Special Care Dentistry

Editor

BURTON S. WASSERMAN

DENTAL CLINICS OF NORTH AMERICA

www.dental.theclinics.com

July 2016 • Volume 60 • Number 3

ELSEVIER

1600 John F. Kennedy Boulevard • Suite 1800 • Philadelphia, Pennsylvania, 19103-2899

http://www.dental.theclinics.com

DENTAL CLINICS OF NORTH AMERICA Volume 60, Number 3
July 2016 ISSN 0011-8532, ISBN: 978-0-323-44843-7

Editor: John Vassallo; j.vassallo@elsevier.com
Developmental Editor: Kristen Helm

Dental Clinics of North America (ISSN 0011-8532) is published quarterly by Elsevier Inc., 360 Park Avenue South, New York, NY 10010-1710. Months of issue are January, April, July, and October. Business and Editorial Offices: 1600 John F. Kennedy Boulevard, Suite 1800, Philadelphia, PA 19103-2899. Periodicals postage paid at New York, NY and additional mailing offices. Subscription prices are $280.00 per year (domestic individuals), $537.00 per year (domestic institutions), $100.00 per year (domestic students/residents), $340.00 per year (Canadian individuals), $695.00 per year (Canadian institutions), $410.00 per year (international individuals), $695.00 per year (international institutions), and $200.00 per year (international and Canadian students/residents). International air speed delivery is included in all *Clinics* subscription prices. All prices are subject to change without notice. **POSTMASTER:** Send address changes to *Dental Clinics of North America*, Elsevier Health Sciences Division, Subscription Customer Service, 3251 Riverport Lane, Maryland Heights, MO 63043. **Customer Service (orders, claims, online, change of address): Elsevier Health Sciences Division, Subscription Customer Service, 3251 Riverport Lane, Maryland Heights, MO 63043. Tel: 1-800-654-2452 (U.S. and Canada). Fax: 314-447-8029. E-mail: journalscustomer service-usa@elsevier.com (for print support); journalsonlinesupport-usa@elsevier.com (for online support).**

Reprints. For copies of 100 or more, of articles in this publication, please contact the Commercial Reprints Department, Elsevier Inc., 360 Park Avenue South, New York, NY 10010-1710. Tel.: 212-633-3874; Fax: 212-633-3820; E-mail: reprints@elsevier.com.

The Dental Clinics of North America is covered in *MEDLINE/PubMed (Index Medicus), Current Contents/Clinical Medicine, ISI/BIOMED* and *Clinahl*.

Contributors

EDITOR

BURTON S. WASSERMAN, DDS, DABSCD
Founding Chairman and Program Director Emeritus, Department of Dental and Oral Medicine, New York-Presbyterian/Queens, Flushing, New York; Former Chairman, Committee for Network Dental Services, New York-Presbyterian Heath Care System, New York, New York; Clinical Professor of Dentistry, Columbia University School of Dental Medicine, New York, New York; Clinical Professor of Surgery; Weill Medical College of Cornell University, New York, New York; Clinical Professor of Dentistry, SUNY Stony Brook School of Dental Medicine, Stony Brook, New York; Associate Professor of Dentistry, NYU College of Dentistry, New York, New York; Adjunct Professor of Dental Medicine, New York Medical College, Valhalla, New York; Private Practice, Flushing, New York

AUTHORS

LISA V. BUDA, DDS
Chief Dental Director, The Blende Dental Group; Department of Surgery, Dental Division, California Pacific Medical Center; Department of Surgery, Dental Division, Kaiser Permanente, San Francisco, California

DAVID B. CLARK, DDS, MSc, FRCDC
Director, Dental Services, Ontario Shores Centre for Mental Health Sciences, Whitby, Ontario, Canada

KIMBERLY M. ESPINOZA, DDS, MPH
Director, Dental Education in the Care of Persons with Disabilities Program; Clinical Assistant Professor, Department of Oral Medicine, University of Washington School of Dentistry, Seattle, Washington

LISA J. HEATON, PhD
Clinical Assistant Professor, Department of Oral Health Sciences, University of Washington School of Dentistry, Seattle, Washington

HARVEY LEVY, DMD, MAGD, DABSCD
Proprietor of Dr Harvey Levy and Associates, PC; Active Staff Member, Department of Surgery, Frederick Memorial Hospital, Frederick, Maryland

AZIZAH BIN MUBAYRIK, BDS, MSc, Clin Cert.
Department Oral Medicine and Diagnostic Sciences, College of Dentistry, King Saud University, Riyadh, Saudi Arabia

ALAN N. QUEEN, DDS, FAGD
Director of Special Needs Dentistry and Attending Dentist, Department of Dental and Oral Medicine, NewYork Presbyterian/Queens Medical Center, Flushing, New York; Private Practice, Flushing, New York

MIRIAM R. ROBBINS, DDS, MS
Department of Dental Medicine, Winthrop University Hospital, Mineola, New York

LENA R. ROTENBERG, MS, MEd
Director of Impossible Projects, Dr Harvey Levy and Associates, PC, Frederick, Maryland

CRAIG C. SPANGLER, DDS, FSCDA
Chief, Division of Dentistry and Oral and Maxillofacial Surgery, Director of the General Practice Residency in Dentistry, St Joseph Mercy Oakland, Pontiac, Michigan; Private Practice of General Dentistry, Bloomfield Hills, Michigan

STANLEY R. SURABIAN, DDS, JD, FACD, FICD, DABSCD
Community Medical Centers' Chief of Dental Services and Program Director of the General Practice Residency in Dentistry, Community Regional Medical Center, Surabian Dental Care Center, Fresno, California

ANNETTA KIT LAM TSANG, BDSc(Hons), GCClinDent, GCEd(HE), MScMed (Pain Mgt), DClinDent (Paed Dent), PhD
Dental Specialist, Pediatric Dentistry, Gold Coast Oral Health Service, Gold Coast University Hospital, Southport, Queensland, Australia; Adjunct Associate Professor, Griffith Health, Griffith University, Queensland, Australia

CHARLES ZAHEDI, DDS, PhD
Department of Periodontics, University of California, Los Angeles (UCLA), Implant Mentoring/Implant Outreach Institute, Newport Beach, California

Contents

Mental Health Issues and Special Care Patients   551

David B. Clark

> Mental illness is a major health issue in the world today, yet often remains misunderstood, unrecognized, and undertreated. Patients suffering from severe psychiatric disorders generally display poor oral health, often as a consequence of both lifestyle and avoidant-type behaviors that become exacerbated by their illness. Individuals with severe mental illness display a greater incidence of oral disease compared with a similar demographic not dealing with these particular disorders. Efforts to enhance the oral health of these vulnerable patients will play a significant role in the overall rebuilding of their self-esteem and contribute positively to their journey toward stability and recovery.

Tools and Equipment for Managing Special Care Patients Anywhere   567

Harvey Levy and Lena R. Rotenberg

> This article describes many of the tools and equipment used by dental professionals to successfully treat special care patients in a variety of settings. Such equipment can be used in the dental office, operating room, hospital, surgical center, nursing home, private home, institution, hospice, and even in the field without electricity. Equipment discussed includes seating, laughing gas and sedation systems, body wraps and mouth props, lighting, radiographic exposure and imaging systems, dental isolation devices, and other tools the authors use.

Ensuring Maintenance of Oral Hygiene in Persons with Special Needs   593

Lisa V. Buda

> Patients with special needs often must rely on inadequately trained caregivers for oral health maintenance. Consequently, full compliance is often not achieved. It is crucial that dentists carefully consider restorative materials and restoration design to maximize durability and facilitate cleansing in these challenging circumstances. This article discusses materials selection, prosthetic design, and oral hygiene techniques for caregivers to ensure longevity and maintenance of oral health in the special needs population.

Evidence-based Dentistry and Its Role in Caring for Special Needs Patients   605

Alan N. Queen

> Evidence-based dentistry is a concept ideally suited and applicable to special needs dentistry. As the special needs of patients varies according

to the individual, so should the way we evaluate our patient, prescribe a course of treatment, and implement that treatment plan. Future generations of dental students and residents should be trained in these concepts not just for patients with special needs, but also for the general patient population. It is imperative that the dental community not retreat in the face of what many deem to be "difficult" patients with special needs. Knowledge and training can overcome many barriers to treatment.

Down syndrome is a common disorder with many oral conditions and systemic manifestations. Dentists need to take a holistic approach including behavioral, oral, and systemic issues. This review of the literature focuses on oral anomalies, systemic interaction, management, and recommendations.

This article focuses on understanding the Americans with Disabilities Act and developmental disabilities for health care providers in special care dentistry. Essential to this awareness is a comprehension of statutory and regulatory requirements and how state disability acts can be more rigorous in application. Developmental disabilities are re-examined in the context of the *Diagnostic and Statistical Manual of Mental Disorders* (Fifth Edition). Understanding of intellectual disability, epilepsy, autism spectrum disorder, and cerebral palsy is necessary because the management of oral health considerations for special care patients has become ever more complex and indispensable.

Today many young dentists want to find a way to make their practices satisfying in ways other than the financial rewards of dentistry. Some of these practitioners have gained additional training in diagnosis and treatment of medically and physically compromised patients in hospital-based, general practice residency programs. A hospital affiliation can create a unique niche that will allow dentists to differentiate themselves from other dentists. By welcoming those ongoing relationships for patients with special needs, and having the resources and desire to treat them, dentists will achieve greater visibility and a reputation as caring, capable practitioners in their community.

The oral handicap of complete edentulism is the terminal outcome of a multifactorial process involving biological factors and patient-related factors. Fully edentulous orally handicapped older adults have been neglected because removable acrylic dentures have been the classic therapy for complete edentulism but are only rehabilitative, not therapeutic. Not replacing missing teeth with stable dentures could prevent adequate food intake. Osseointegrated endosseous implants used as a therapeutic adjunct can reduce the problem of long-term bone resorption to less than 0.1 mm per year. Implant-borne prostheses substantially increase the overall health and quality of life of orally handicapped fully edentulous older adults.

Communicating with Patients with Special Health Care Needs 693

Kimberly M. Espinoza and Lisa J. Heaton

People with special health care needs (PSHCN) often have difficulty communicating with providers in health care settings, including dental practices. This difficulty can affect access to care as well as the quality of care received. This article provides practical tips and tools dental professionals can use to facilitate communication for a diverse population of PSHCNs. The article discusses communication needs of patients with communication disorders; augmentative and alternative communication; and communication for patients with intellectual disability, psychiatric conditions; and dental fears. Examples are given of communication breakdowns, and descriptions of how communication challenges can be resolved.

Neurologic Diseases in Special Care Patients 707

Miriam R. Robbins

Neurologic diseases can have a major impact on functional capacity. Patients with neurologic disease require individualized management considerations depending on the extent of impairment and impact on functional capacity. This article reviews 4 of the more common and significant neurologic diseases (Alzheimer disease, cerebrovascular accident/stroke, multiple sclerosis, and Parkinson disease) that are likely to present to a dental office and provides suggestions on the dental management of patients with these conditions.

The Special Needs of Preterm Children – An Oral Health Perspective 737

Annetta Kit Lam Tsang

Preterm births are defined as those before 37 weeks of gestation. With advances in fertility medicine and neonatal medicine, the numbers of preterm children in the community have significantly increased. Developmental delays and complications among preterm children are well recognized. Much less consideration is given to the dental complications of preterm children. Manifestations include palatal deformations, enamel defects, tooth size variations and tooth shape deformities, malocclusions, and increased risks of early childhood caries and tooth wear. This article explores orodental risks and orodental needs of preterm children and suggests preventive and management strategies for optimizing the oral health of special needs children.

DENTAL CLINICS OF NORTH AMERICA

Dedication

It is an honor to dedicate this issue to both the special needs patients who often are in dire need of dental treatment and the providers who willingly sacrifice their time and clinical expertise to manage these patients.

Burton S. Wasserman, DDS, DABSCD
55-14 Main Street
Flushing, NY 11355, USA

E-mail address:
bswasser@nyp.org

Preface

Special Care Dentistry

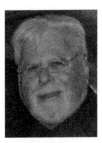

Burton S. Wasserman, DDS, DABSCD
Editor

The subject of Special Care Dentistry has received significant notoriety during the past 7 years. Dental schools have responded very positively by increasing their Special Care curricula. Hospital general practice and pediatric residency programs have dedicated special needs as part of the resident's didactic and clinical experiences. The national organization "Special Care in Dentistry Association" has expanded its mission by emphasizing the treatment options for the special needs patient.

There have been worthwhile discussions related to considering special needs dentistry as a recognized Commission on Dental Accreditation specialty.

Mr John Vassallo, the editor of *Dental Clinics of North America*, and Ms Kristen Helm, the developmental editor, have been extremely helpful in establishing the parameters for a readable and well-sequenced text. The primary goals in preparing this issue include access to care, disease entities, and treatment methodologies. We applaud the authors who have dedicated their time and writing skills as well as sharing their professional experiences. The result is an outstanding and informative issue of *Dental Clinics of North America* focused on the oral health needs of special needs patients. Of course, I am extremely grateful to my dear wife and partner, Dr June Wasserman, my loving and supportive children and grandchildren, and my office coordinator, Victoria Giordano.

I was fortunate to have been the editor of "The Special Care Patient" (*Dental Clinics of North America*, April 2009). This current issue (July 2016) addresses the needs of special care patients in a changing environment where the dental profession has stepped forward to expand the Special Care curricula in dental schools and encourage

Dent Clin N Am 60 (2016) xi–xii
http://dx.doi.org/10.1016/j.cden.2016.03.003
0011-8532/16/$ – see front matter © 2016 Published by Elsevier Inc.

dental.theclinics.com

recent dental graduates to be comfortable in treating this often forgotten and under-served population.

Burton S. Wasserman, DDS, DABSCD
Department of Dental and Oral Medicine
New York-Presbyterian/Queens
Flushing, NY 11355, USA

New York-Presbyterian Heath Care System
New York, NY, USA

Columbia University School
of Dental Medicine
New York, NY, USA

Weill Medical College
of Cornell University
New York, NY, USA

SUNY Stony Brook School of Dental Medicine
Stony Brook, NY, USA

NYU College of Dentistry
New York, NY, USA

New York Medical College
Valhalla, NY, USA

Private Practice
55-14 Main Street
Flushing, NY 11355, USA

E-mail address:
bswasser@nyp.org

Mental Health Issues and Special Care Patients

David B. Clark, DDS, MSc, FRCDC*

KEYWORDS

- Mental illness • Psychotropic medications • Stigma • Oral health complications
- Xerostomia • Addictions

KEY POINTS

- Patients with mental health issues bring unique needs and differing priorities to a dental practice and the dental practitioner must be mindful and flexible of these factors.
- Dentistry can play a significant role in the diagnosis, support, and management of individuals dealing with severe mental illness.
- Effective communication and collaboration between dentists, physicians, psychiatrists, nursing, and social services and the patient's family is essential to promoting effective oral health initiatives and care for those individuals with severe mental health issues.
- Overwhelming evidence has shown that those individuals suffering from severe mental health issues experience enormous disparities rather than advantages in the quality and quantity of health care services.
- Individuals with severe mental illness display a greater incidence of oral disease, including rampant caries, periodontal disease, xerostomia, and tooth loss.

INTRODUCTION

Psychiatric disease and dental disease are viewed as 2 of the most prevalent health problems that exist in society today. Approximately 1 in 5 people in North America will suffer from some form of psychiatric illness at some point during their lifetime.[1,2] Depression, the most common mental illness, is estimated to become the second leading cause of disability worldwide by 2020, second only to ischemic cardiovascular disease.[3]

Mental illness can include such disorders as schizophrenia and other forms of psychoses, anxiety disorders, eating disorders, mood disorders (eg, depression, bipolar affective disorder), and personality disorders. A specific diagnosis is made on the

Disclosure Statement: The author has no commercial or financial conflicts of interest and has no funding sources in preparing this article.
Dental Services, Ontario Shores Centre for Mental Health Sciences, 700 Gordon Street, Whitby, Ontario L1N 5S9, Canada
* 74 Martindale Street, Oshawa, Ontario L1H 6W6, Canada.
E-mail address: davidclark1461@gmail.com

Dent Clin N Am 60 (2016) 551–566
http://dx.doi.org/10.1016/j.cden.2016.02.001
0011-8532/16/$ – see front matter © 2016 Elsevier Inc. All rights reserved.

dental.theclinics.com

basis of a cluster of particular symptoms, each with a clinical significance or impairment criterion. It is this methodology that comprises the *Diagnostic and Statistical Manual of Mental Disorders, Fifth Edition* (DSM-V), which is the standard reference for defining and classifying psychiatric disease in North America.[4] Despite twentieth century advances in disease diagnosis and treatment, the concept of a distinction between mental illness and physical illness has persisted in our perception and dialogue surrounding disease. This misconception surrounding the separation of mind and body along with a further separation of mental health treatment from mainstream medical care has provided significant impetus to the stigmatization of people suffering from psychiatric illness.[5–7] Results of a Canadian national health survey in 2008 highlight the public's perception of mental illness revealing some startling, and yet not surprising views on this devastating group of diseases.[8] The survey results are summarized in **Box 1**.

A significant and yet often unspoken barrier to accessing much-needed oral care is the misconception held by not only health care professionals but the public at large, that those individuals dealing with issues of mental illness are inherently unpredictable and, therefore, dangerous and violent toward others. The reality is that fewer than 4% of violent criminal acts can be attributed to someone with a history of mental illness in contrast to that portion of violent criminal activity in the community at large.[1,9,10] Unfortunately, one single case of violence (combined with heightened media portrayals) can undermine any progress being made to fight stigma and discrimination against this most vulnerable segment of society. This misconception also serves to undermine the reality that individuals with severe mental illness will be of more harm to themselves or will in fact be the victims of criminal violence.[10]

Mental illness is an "equal opportunity disease," affecting people of all ages, all races, and all educational backgrounds and economic groups (**Fig. 1**).[11,12]

Up to two-thirds of individuals suffering from various signs and symptoms of a severe mental illness will not receive a proper and timely diagnosis with appropriate follow-up treatment. Stigma is generally cited as the main formidable barrier to care.[5] Coping strategies often used in lieu of seeking professional treatment include such negative behaviors as denial and substance abuse.[5] Stigmatization of individuals with severe mental health issues has persisted throughout history and is exemplified by distrust, fear, bias, stereotyping, embarrassment, and often avoidance. In turn, this complicates and even reduces a person's ability to access resources and opportunities for treatment. The end result often leads to low self-esteem, isolation, and a sense of hopelessness. A tragic and yet preventable result of this long-term disease is suicide. As health care professionals, dental practitioners must play a vital role in

---

Box 1
Survey results among Canadians regarding stigma toward mental illness

46% of respondents believe mental illness is used as an excuse for bad behavior

25% of respondents fear to be around those with mental illness

50% of respondents would disclose their relationship with someone with mental illness versus

72% for someone with cancer; 68% for someone with diabetes

50% of respondents view alcohol/drug addictions as not being mental illnesses

Data from National Report Card on Health Care. Canadian Medical Association, 2008. Available at: http://www.cbc.ca/health/story/2008/08/15/mental-health.html. Accessed September 15, 2015.

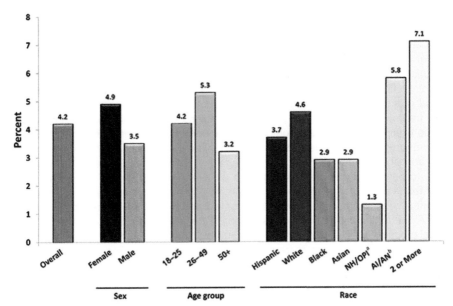

Fig. 1. Prevalence of serious mental illness among US adults (2013). AI, American Indian; AN, Alaska Native; NH, Native Hawaiian; OPI, Other Pacific Islander. (*From* National Institute of Mental Health (NIMH). Serious Mental Illness (SMI) among U.S. adults. Available at: https://www.nimh.nih.gov/health/statistics/prevalence/serious-mental-illness-smi-among-us-adults.shtml. Accessed October 15, 2015; with permission.)

helping to deprogram this stereotypical approach with not only their peers, but patients alike suffering from severe mental illness and, alternatively, exhibit more sensitivity to the innumerable vulnerability factors and potential psychological problems inherent in this patient population.

Although both oral and dental problems are similar between those with or without serious mental health issues, evidence strongly suggests that those individuals with serious mental illness display a greater risk of oral disease resulting in an even greater need for treatment.[2,13,14] Some of the factors that are deemed to impact the oral health and the access and provision of oral care for those dealing with serious mental health problems include the following:

- Type, severity, and stage of mental illness
- Mood, motivation, and self-esteem
- Lack of perception of oral health problems
- Habits, lifestyle, and ability to sustain self-care and dental attendance
- Side effects of medication
- Overcoming barriers to oral health care

TYPE, SEVERITY, AND STAGE OF MENTAL ILLNESS

Mental illness is regarded as a chronic disease that, in many instances, tends to fluctuate in terms of symptomatology depending on the specific diagnosis (eg, bipolar affective disorder), as well as individual responses to medications and psychotherapy, including the availability of support systems (eg, family, friends). In some situations, oral symptoms may be the first presenting feature identified by the dental practitioner of an underlying mental health problem. Excessive enamel erosion (often seen within

6 months of the onset of frequent purging behavior in bulimia),[15,16] unexplained facial or temporomandibular joint pain,[17] and self-inflicted oral trauma[18,19] are a few of these initial oral symptoms that may be experienced by the individual dealing with severe mental illness.

A prior history of sexual abuse is a frequent predictor of future mental health issues, including mood disorders, eating disorders, and substance abuse problems.[20,21] Dental practitioners will also treat patients who have experienced a wide range of other traumatic life experiences in addition to episodes of sexual abuse, including domestic violence, elder abuse, combat trauma, and other traumatic life events (eg, 9/11).[22] Short-term consequences of traumatic experiences can include mistrust, anxiety, and social isolation, which if undiagnosed and untreated, lead, in the long term, to negative coping strategies such as overeating, smoking, alcoholism, and other forms of substance abuse. In addition, victims of trauma will likely avoid seeking out either routine preventive medical or dental care. Individuals often experience difficulty in adapting to the close physical space contact inherent in otherwise routine dental procedures. The development of comorbidities such as anxiety and depression can contribute, for example, to frequent canceling and rescheduling of dental appointments. Consequently, many years may pass during which the individual avoids seeking proper oral health care services, often resulting in a more rapid deterioration of both the teeth and supporting structures. This deterioration is further exacerbated by the side effects of prescribed medications, as well as the deleterious effects of prolonged substance abuse. Patients suffering from a long-term addictive illness may present with behavioral, nutritional, and social changes, as well as demonstrating early impairment of cognitive functioning. Chronic substance abuse often results in depression, lack of motivation, and decreased self-image, adversely impacting oral health care. The effects of street drugs, such as methamphetamines, cocaine, and ecstasy, have all been well documented in the dental literature as to the devastating consequences involving the teeth, periodontium, and oral mucosa, as well as a heightened potential for trauma and dentofacial injury.[2,23,24]

Patients who have been diagnosed as suffering from a somatoform disorder may present with complaints of physical symptoms suggestive of a physical disorder but for which there is no demonstrable underlying physical basis.[2,25] Body dysmorphic disorder represents one subtype of somatoform disorder whereby the individual develops a preoccupation with an exaggerated defect in some aspect of his or her physical appearance. This condition may affect up to 25% of the population and may be one of the key underlying causes of patient dissatisfaction with certain physical or dental features, such as facial asymmetry, or a disproportion of shape and size involving, for example, the lips and jaws or the appearance of the teeth. The dental practitioner must show increased vigilance to the potential presence of disproportionate concerns surrounding appearance, particularly in planning comprehensive esthetic treatment plans.[26]

Obsessive compulsive disorder (OCD) is a form of anxiety disorder whereby individuals will describe the presence of intrusive, preoccupying thoughts that make them anxious and upset. Such obsessive thoughts can be unwanted and trivial, or may often be highly charged, and the individual will carry out compulsive or repetitive behaviors (most commonly cleaning and checking) to allay their anxiety. Such compulsive behavior begins to dominate a person's life interfering with day-to-day activities including relationships and work leading to embarrassment, further anxiety, and often depression.[27] Oral manifestations may include overzealous oral hygiene practices (eg, tooth brushing, prolonged use of mouthwashes) that may lead to excessive tooth or soft tissue trauma.

Eating disorders (eg, anorexia, bulimia, binge-eating disorder) represent a serious, life-threatening illness affecting a disproportionate number of females, often arising during early adolescence.[28,29] The lifetime prevalence is approximately 1.5% to 2.0%. Although food appears to be the central issue, it is really the characterization of food-related problems that become an outlet for the expression of a variety of more serious underlying psychological issues. The result becomes a problematic coping strategy. Dieting quickly becomes a measure of self-esteem giving the individual a sense of personal control resulting in an ongoing obsession with weight loss, food, and exercise. Such a change in focus perpetuates the illness with potentially severe consequences. The mind develops a distorted or even delusional thought process around body image, perceiving oneself as continually being too fat. Psychopathology quickly translates into a physiopathology defining a particular subtype of eating disorder. Oral manifestations of eating disorders can impair oral function, cause pain, and lead to a deterioration of esthetics and quality of life[30] (**Table 1**).

MOOD, MOTIVATION, AND SELF-ESTEEM

Researchers have suggested that those individuals diagnosed with depression may display a higher propensity for physical illness, largely through the negative effects on the immune system potentially leading to a greater risk for infection.[31] Patients who experience major depressive episodes will often show a total disregard for maintaining any daily oral hygiene care. Salivary gland output may decrease and, along with an increased consumption of carbohydrates and increased lactobacillus count, patients will display a greater tendency for increased caries and periodontal disease.[32] Patients experiencing either the manic or hypomanic phase of bipolar disorder may exhibit more aggressive tendencies in terms of performing daily oral hygiene procedures, causing, for example, excessive abrasion lesions to the teeth, with or without gingival lacerations.[2,33–35]

Schizophrenia represents the most common and serious form of psychotic illness that affects mood, thought, and behavior and for which there remains no cure.[36] Individuals in essence, lose touch with reality, becoming increasingly unsure whether their thoughts and experiences are real or not. Such thought disturbances and aberrant behaviors, in turn, reduce the ability of an individual to maintain self-care as well as to be

Table 1
Oral manifestations of eating disorders

Location	Findings	Etiology
Teeth	Erosion; caries; thermal sensitivity; chipping of teeth; anterior open bite	Vomiting; poor oral hygiene; high carbohydrate intake
Mucosal lesions	Mucosal atrophy; glossodynia; glossitis; erythema (soft palate); dysgeusia	Vitamin deficiency (eg, B6, B12); vomiting; nutritional deficiency
Periodontal lesions	Gingivitis; periodontitis	Vitamin deficiency (eg, vitamin C); poor oral hygiene
Salivary changes	Enlargement of major/minor salivary glands (sialadenosis); xerostomia	Metabolic/secretory abnormalities; concurrent medications; for example, antidepressants

From Clark DB. Patients with eating disorders: challenges for the oral health professional. Can J Dent Hyg 2010;44(4):167; with permission.

able to maintain meaningful social and work relationships. Individuals diagnosed with schizophrenia or other forms of acute psychoses may display a varying predominance of positive, negative, or disorganized symptoms inherent within the disease itself[2,37,38] (**Table 2**).

These various symptoms in turn may be accompanied by varying degrees of cognitive impairment and social or occupational dysfunction. In particular, the negative symptom complex of this disease (absence of emotion, social detachment, lack of expression, lack of motivation and initiative) is associated more with the long-term chronicity of the disease, and can impact on one's ability to think logically and be able to understand, accept, and cooperate with a plan of routine dental care. The lack of motivation or apathy to perform activities of normal daily living, including oral care is unfortunately often misconstrued by others as simple laziness.

Symptoms associated with more acute forms of psychotic illness (eg, delusional or paranoid ideation) will often affect the acceptance of dental treatment leading to extended periods of neglect. This often results in a pattern of rampant decay with or without periodontal disease usually diagnosed at such a time that full mouth extractions are often inevitable.

Delusional thoughts may focus directly on the oral cavity. Suspicions may be aroused that restorations placed into one's teeth may in fact contain tiny transmitters, further enhancing feelings of thought broadcasting, though insertion, and so forth.[2] Acts of orofacial and self-mutilation have also been described in the literature, particularly in those individuals at the height of an acute psychotic episode. These acts have included multiple autoextractions,[18] glossectomy,[39] self-enucleation of the eye,[40] excoriation of gingival tissues with sharp fingernails, and burning of the gingivae with caustic substances.[41]

The progression of dementia, particularly in the elderly population, invariably carries with it a progressive decline in self-care (including oral care) unless a familiar caregiver has been involved in the very early stages of the disease to learn to provide these services on a regular basis during the terminal part of the illness.[42–44] Dementia is also

Table 2		
Symptomatology of schizophrenia		
Positive Symptoms: Behaviors that *Should* Not Be Present	**Negative Symptoms: Absences of Behavior that *Should* Be Present**	**Disorganized Symptoms**
Exaggeration of ideas and thoughts (grandiose) Delusions: persecutory type, thought broadcasting, thought insertion, thought withdrawal, being controlled by others Hallucinations: auditory("voices"), visual, tactile, somatic	Disturbances of affect: flat emotion, lack of expression, monotony of speech Impaired interpersonal relationships Lack of motivation, apathy, social withdrawal Absence of normal drives/ interest including self-care = poor general/oral hygiene(dental caries, periodontal disease, loss of teeth)	Thought disturbances: rapid shift of ideas, poor thought relation, incoherent speech Bizarre behavior: ritualistic, stereotypical, gesturing, imitating speech of others, mutism, pacing

From Clark DB. Dental care for the patient with schizophrenia. Can J Dent Hyg 2008;42(1):19; with permission.

often associated with other psychological comorbidities, including anxiety and depression. It is not surprising therefore that a progressive decline in oral care, combined with other factors, such as dry mouth secondary to medications, will predominate with an inevitable decline in self-esteem. Unfortunately, it is often mistakenly believed that the individual is no longer capable of experiencing such an emotion because of his or her overlying psychiatric illness.

LACK OF PERCEPTION OF ORAL HEALTH PROBLEMS

Preventive dental education remains a critical aspect of the dental management protocol for patients suffering from a variety of psychiatric illnesses. In light of the episodic and recurrent nature of many of these diseases (eg, bipolar affective disorder), the dental practitioner must be capable of applying some modification to any oral care treatment regimens.

Behavioral factors associated with severe mental illness can result in poor compliance coupled with unreliable attendance and late cancellation of dental appointments. Irregular attendance is often fueled by fear, anxiety, and lack of consistent financial resources or support. Noncompliance to prescribed dental care often mirrors a noncompliant attitude to medical care in general, and it is these negative perceptions of need on the part of the patient that will present the most challenges to the dental practitioner. Lack of understanding or insight into a specific mental illness, and the sometimes intolerable side effects of medications, can contribute to the high rate of noncompliance with psychopharmacotherapy. If the patient is unable or unwilling to believe that oral health needs are important, the oral health will quickly suffer and the efforts of a dental practitioner become severely compromised.[14] Understanding the symptoms status, functional status, and level of health needs perception of the individual allows for the dental practitioner to understand more fully the individual's capacity for changing oral health behaviors at any given time during the course of the illness. There is, therefore, a requirement on the part of the dental practitioner for flexibility and pragmatism in terms of the capacity and motivation of the patient toward obtaining oral health care. Oral hygiene practices may, for example, vary from complete cooperation at one appointment to partial or total lack of participation at another visit based on the symptom status that the patient exhibits each time. The lack of perception of the existence of any oral health problems may necessitate more frequent appointment scheduling or other treatment modifications, particularly for those patients suffering from moderate to severe xerostomia secondary to psychotropic medications.[2,34,45] Engaging the support of family members to ensure some form of adherence to daily oral hygiene practice is another viable management strategy.

PATIENT'S HABITS, LIFESTYLE, AND ABILITY TO SUSTAIN SELF-CARE AND DENTAL ATTENDANCE

Individuals diagnosed with a serious mental illness often experience a double-burden with their illness that includes not only the signs and symptoms associated with a specific psychiatric diagnosis but also the coexisting stigma and discrimination that create barriers to one's ability to gain the necessary knowledge on how to access needed health care resources to effect treatment and change. This may further exacerbate an already compromised quality of life and lead to diminished self-esteem, isolation, and a sense of hopelessness, all of which can provide fertile ground for other comorbid behaviors such as increased substance abuse. This cycle becomes self-perpetuating in a very short period of time. For example, the reported incidence of alcohol abuse in patients with bipolar disorder can be as high as 44% compared with less than 17% of the general population.[46] This comorbidity of addiction can result in increased challenges for medical treatment, a greater incidence of suicidal ideation, and potential increase in completing an act of suicide.

The onset of schizophrenia is often in early adulthood at a time when individuals are pursuing postsecondary educational opportunities, or embarking on a newly chosen career path. The delay of such pursuits in schizophrenia impacts significantly on their level of independence, both financial and otherwise. Failure of individuals suffering from schizophrenia to access needed dental care may be due in part to[2] the following:

- A lack of motivation to perform daily oral hygiene care
- Inability to plan
- Feelings of stigmatization by health care professionals in general
- The potential orofacial side effects of many psychotropic medications used in treatment today

Dental patients are often reluctant to disclose a current or past history of psychiatric care largely out of the stigma and embarrassment that they feel.[6,7] It is often easier to talk to a patient about the symptoms or management of their diabetes, for example, than it is about mental health issues. The dental practitioner must maintain a level of sensitivity and empathy to a patient's vulnerability factors and psychological problems to be able to provide as consistently as possible the highest quality of dental care for that particular patient. The approach of the dental practitioner must be designed to obtain as much information as possible about the severity of the disorder (as opposed to just the diagnosis), the treatments the patient is receiving, and the effectiveness of these interventions (**Box 2**).

Mortality data indicate that those patients who suffer from a serious mental health disorder (eg, schizophrenia, bipolar disorder, major depression) will die, on average, 25 years earlier than the general population.[47–50] This shortened life span is not directly attributable to increased rates of suicide or accidents but rather to the increased rates of ischemic heart disease, type 2 diabetes, respiratory illness, and cancer stemming from the higher incidence of such risk factors as hypertension, obesity, and alterations in both glucose and fat metabolism seen much more frequently in this vulnerable patient population.[51–53] These risk factors arise largely from medication side effects as well as the significant lifestyle differences inherent in those who suffer from severe mental illness. This cluster of physical risk factors is referred to as "metabolic syndrome." Metabolic syndrome, as defined by the International Diabetes Federation,[54] is the presence of visceral obesity (waist circumference criteria) accompanied by any 2 of the following factors: hypertriglyceridemia, reduced high-density lipoprotein (HDL) cholesterol levels, hypertension, and raised fasting glycemia (type 2 diabetes). A marked increase in such modifiable risk factors as smoking, alcohol consumption,

---

Box 2
Questions that may be used to help expand on a patient's mental health history

1. When was your mental illness diagnosed?

2. What medications are you taking for management of your illness (eg, antidepressants, antipsychotics, antianxiety agents)?

3. How long have you been taking the medications? Do they help you?

4. Have you experienced any oral side effects, such as dry mouth, burning tongue, excessive saliva, or swollen gums?

5. Who is the general practitioner/psychiatrist treating your illness?

"unsafe" sexual behaviors, poor nutrition, obesity, and substance abuse coupled with inadequate access to health care services also serve to heighten the risk of morbidity and mortality in this vulnerable population. The oral-systemic paradigm becomes increasingly relevant in this patient population, focusing not only on the systemic complications linked to oral inflammation and infection but also to the oral manifestations of systemic disease.[55]

Epidemiologic studies have described such oral diseases as periodontal disease, caries, hyposalivation, and edentulousness as being associated with most features of metabolic syndrome.[56] The relationship of diabetes and cardiovascular disease to one's oral health has become increasingly theorized, with various physiologic mechanisms proposed to understand more fully the underlying inflammatory mechanisms common to both and has increasingly been the subject of the debate around the oral-systemic health paradigm.

For example, the level of obesity is described as being closely aligned with the state of one's oral health, specifically, the severity of periodontal disease, caries, and hyposalivation; any of which oral findings may contribute to eventual tooth loss.[57] Metabolic syndrome has also been postulated as an independent risk factor for periodontal disease with obesity and its associated proinflammatory state being evaluated as one major factor facilitating this relationship.[55,58]

Between 50% and 80% of patients suffering from severe mental health issues smoke compared with approximately 25% of the general population.[59] Not only can this contribute to increased rates of lung cancer in this vulnerable population but it also heightens the potential for oral cancer, particular in combination with alcohol abuse. Smoking can present significant difficulty for the medical practitioner to titrate effective blood levels of some antipsychotics, such as olanzapine and clozapine, largely due to competition involving the liver metabolism of these drugs.[60] Other deleterious oral effects from smoking can include an increased incidence of periodontal disease, candidiasis, and xerostomia. Increased vigilance on the part of the dental professional is required as part of a routine head and neck examination whenever opportunistic screening is available.

SIDE EFFECTS OF MEDICATION

Along with the various modalities of psychotherapy and skills training, pharmacotherapy remains a cornerstone for the stabilization and long-term management of most psychiatric illnesses. As with many of the medications that dental patients might be taking, psychotropic medications can also have significant side effects that can clearly manifest within the oral cavity.[2,61–63] Xerostomia remains the most common and frequently reported side effect. The prevalence varies by drug and concomitant use of other medications, which may create a cumulative effect for the development of dry mouth. Xerostomia can have significant deleterious consequences including the following[2,64–67]:

- Increased incidence of caries (especially root caries)
- Gingivitis
- Stomatitis
- Oral ulceration
- Dysphagia
- Burning mouth
- Diminished taste acuity
- Difficulty chewing and speaking
- Increased susceptibility to candidal infections.

Attempts by patients to counteract oral dryness often include an increased intake of candies or chewing gum with or without a greater consumption of sweetened soda drinks or juices.

Denture wearers will also experience greater difficulty in retaining and wearing complete dentures comfortably. This can impact secondarily on their overall nutritional status as well as self-esteem and social interactions. Protocols aimed at reducing the subjective feelings of dry mouth as well as providing preventive oral care must now be part of a dental practitioner's armamentarium when planning denture treatment.[2,66,68]

Drug-induced orofacial movement disorders or oral dyskinesias are represented by abnormal involuntary movements that may vary both in severity and distribution dependent on the drug dose and duration of therapy.[69] One subtype, tardive dyskinesia, is a long-term complication seen in approximately 25% of patients undergoing treatment with some of the early antipsychotic drugs such as chlorpromazine and haloperidol.[2,37,38] The incidence of such movement disorders has decreased somewhat with the more widespread use of the so-called atypical antipsychotics such as olanzapine, risperidone, quetiapine, ziprasidone, and clozapine, but may still develop as a long-term side effect of treatment. Facial grimacing, lip smacking, jerky tongue movements, and generalized head and neck tremors can comprise some of the main features of tardive dyskinesia and depending on severity, may significantly impact the provision of dental care.

Clozapine is the only atypical antipsychotic medication that carries a 1% risk of agranulocytosis (white blood cell count <3000/mm^3) and, as such, the dental practitioner must be cognizant of such signs and symptoms indicative of infection, including fever, pain, and oral ulceration.[2]

Patients must undergo regular monitoring of their white blood cell count and the dental practitioner needs to be aware of these test results during ongoing dental treatment. In contrast to the predominant side effect of xerostomia, nearly one-third of patients taking clozapine will frequently complain of drooling or sialorrhea, both a stigmatizing and functionally disabling side effect that can affect the individual's compliance in taking the medication. The etiology of this paradoxic side effect that can affect salivary flow is not yet completely understood.[68,70,71]

An increased incidence of both clenching and bruxism has been reported with the use of the selective serotonin reuptake inhibitor (SSRI) class of antidepressants, thought to be a consequence of the effect these drugs have on serotonergic receptors.[17,72–74] Consequently, patients who are identified as exhibiting or complaining of this side effect might be encouraged to wear a night guard appliance to minimize the deleterious effects on the teeth as well as associated temporomandibular joint (TMJ) structures.

The dental practitioner must also be cognizant of significant drug interactions that may occur when used in combination with other nonpsychotropic medications identified in a patient's drug history (**Table 3**).[38]

OVERCOMING BARRIERS TO ORAL HEALTH CARE

Effective communication and collaboration between dentists, physicians, psychiatrists, and nursing and social services and the patient's family is essential in promoting effective oral health care initiatives for those individuals with severe mental health issues. Overwhelming evidence from several studies has shown that those individuals suffering from various psychiatric disorders experience enormous disparities rather than advantages in the quality of health care services and achievement of expected

Table 3
Potential drug interactions involving psychotropic medications

Class of Drug	Interacting Drug	Effect
Neuroleptic (antipsychotic) medications; for example, risperidone, olanzapine, clozapine	Warfarin sodium	• Decreased blood levels of warfarin sodium • Lower International Normalized Ratio (INR) level
	Tricyclic antidepressants	• Increased serum level of both drugs • Marked anticholinergic effect
	Opioid analgesics	• Increased sedative effects of opioids • Increased risk of respiratory depression
	Antihypertensive	• Increased risk of hypotension
	Alcohol	• Increased risk of hypotension • Increased risk of respiratory depression
	Anxiolytics	• Increased risk of sedation • Increased risk of respiratory depression
	Nicotine	• Decreased blood levels of antipsychotics
	Anticonvulsants	• Decreased effects of antipsychotic medications
Antidepressant medications		
a. SSRI	Codeine-containing analgesics	• Reduced analgesic efficacy via effects on P450 hepatic microsomal enzymes
	Warfarin sodium	• Inhibits metabolism of warfarin • Increased INR level
	Sedatives	• Potentiate respiratory depressant effects
b. Tricyclics	Levonordefrin (local anesthetic vasoconstrictor)	• Blocks reuptake of levonordefrin • Marked rise in blood pressure, cardiac dysrhythmias
	Ethanol, opioids, barbiturates	• Potentiate respiratory depressant effects
	Warfarin sodium	• Inhibit metabolism of warfarin • Increased INR level
c. Mood stabilizers (eg, lithium)	Nonsteroidal anti-inflammatory drugs	• Impairs renal excretion of lithium • Potential lithium toxicity • Anticholinergic effect

From Clark DB. Dental care for the patient with schizophrenia. Can J Dent Hyg 2008;42(1):22; with permission.

screening, diagnostic, and treatment benchmarks.[75–78] Among individuals with severe mental illness, oral health care is consistently noted to be poor and an often disregarded health issue.

An oral health assessment must be part of any general health assessment, and dentistry is in a key position to provide leadership in this aspect of total patient care. Dental health practitioners generally see patients on a more frequent basis than their medical colleagues, often over a patient's lifetime, and are therefore in a unique position to foster a closer rapport with their patients. Dental practitioners can therefore be a resource for accessing emergency and specialist services as well as providing preventive advice, including oral health promotion literature and oral hygiene aids and equipment.

Consent may be obtained through established professional guidelines. Patients with mental health issues often bring unique needs and differing priorities to a dental practice, and the dental health practitioner must demonstrate patience, flexibility, empathy, and a nonstigmatizing attitude in caring for these patients. Dental treatment must encompass the concept of rational dental care, whereby patient-focused care is planned after all modifying factors have been assessed (physiologic, psychological, and functional limitations); that is, due diligence has been carried out.

SUMMARY

Psychiatric illness and its medical management carry significant risks for oral disease. Individuals suffering from various mental health issues have not shared over the years in the improvements to the oral health of the general population. Patients with severe mental illness must be entitled to the same standards of oral health care as the remainder of the population and the disparities that have inhibited improved oral health outcomes in this vulnerable patient population must be eliminated.

Understanding the type, severity, and stage of mental illness along with a patient's own mood, motivation, lifestyle, and personal perception of oral disease can enhance the knowledge of the dental professional concerning this critical aspect of a patient's medical history and further illustrates how closely mental health and oral health are intertwined. Dental professionals need to be aware of factors such as reduced rates of compliance with dental treatment (often mirroring that for medical management), reduced ability to access oral health care services, financial restrictions, dental phobias, and the effects of various psychotropic medications on oral health including hyposalivation, caries, and periodontal disease, as well as the potential interactions with drugs used in dental practice.[14]

One of the fundamental tenets of any dental professional-patient relationship is trust, respect, and education, and these factors become no less important in treating patients dealing with severe mental health issues. Dental professionals must strive to maintain a positive, empathetic, and caring attitude: an attitude that is highly correlated to success in an individual's overall rehabilitation and recovery. Enhancing self-esteem and feelings of self-worth for those coping with a severe mental illness can be a very fulfilling experience that can only serve to continue to break down the stigma surrounding this group of diseases.

REFERENCES

1. Brousseau L, Hamel M, Paris J, et al. Report on mental illnesses in Canada. Ottawa (Canada): Public Health Agency of Canada; 2002. Available at: http// www.phac-aspc.gc.ca. Accessed October 15, 2015.
2. Little JW, Falace DA, Miller CS, et al. Neurologic, behavioral, and psychiatric disorders. In: Dental management of the medically compromised patient. 7th edition. St Louis (MO): Mosby Elsevier; 2008. p. 464–507.
3. Murray CJL, Lopez AD. The global burden of disease: a comprehensive assessment of mortality and disability from diseases, injuries, and risk factors in 1990 and projected to 2020. Geneva (Switzerland): World Health Organization; 1996.
4. American Psychiatric Association. Diagnostic and statistical manual of mental disorders, text revision. 5th edition (DSM-V). Washington, DC: American Psychiatric Association; 2013.
5. Mental health: a report of the surgeon general, US Public Health Service. 1999. Available at: http://www.surgeongeneral.gov/library/mentalhealth/home.html. Accessed October 15, 2015.
6. Arboleda-Florez J, Stuart H. From sin to science: fighting the stigmatization of mental illnesses. Can J Psychiatry 2012;57(8):457–63.
7. Stuart H. The stigmatization of mental illnesses. Can J Psychiatry 2012;57(8): 455–6.

8. National report card on health care. Canadian Medical Association; 2008. Available at: http://www.cbc.ca/health/story/2008/08/15/mental-health.html. Accessed September 15, 2015.
9. Simmie S, Nunes J. The last taboo. Toronto: McClelland & Stewart; 2001.
10. Truth versus myth on mental illness, suicide, and crime [Editorial]. Lancet 2013; 382(9901):1309.
11. National Institute of Mental Health (NIMH). Serious Mental Illness (SMI)among U.S. adults. Available at: https://www.nimh.nih.gov/health/statistics/prevalence/serious-mental-illness-smi-among-us-adults.shtml. Accessed October 15, 2015.
12. Kirmayer LJ, Brass GM, Tait CL. The mental health of aboriginal peoples: transformations of identity and community. Can J Psychiatry 2000;45:607–16.
13. Kossioni AE, Kossionis GE, Polychronopoulou A. Oral health status of elderly hospitalized psychiatric patients. Gerodontology 2012;29:272–83.
14. Kisely S, Quek L, Pais J, et al. Advanced dental disease in people with severe mental illness: systematic review and meta-analysis. Br J Psychol 2011;199:187–93.
15. Ashcroft A, Milosevic A. The eating disorders: 1. Current scientific understanding and dental implications. Dent Update 2007;34:544–54.
16. Woodmansey KF. Recognition of bulimia nervosa in dental patients: implications for dental care providers. Gen Dent 2000;48(1):48–51.
17. Winocur E, Hermesh H, Littner D, et al. Signs of bruxism and temporomandibular disorders among psychiatric patients. Oral Surg Oral Med Oral Pathol Oral Radiol Endod 2007;103:60–3.
18. Altom RL, DiAngelos AJ. Multiple autoextractions: oral self-mutilation reviewed. Oral Surg 1989;67:271–4.
19. Hoffman GR, Islam S. Facial trauma patients with a pre-existing psychiatric illness: a 5-year study. Oral Surg Oral Med Oral Pathol Oral Radiol 2013;116:e368–74.
20. Stalker CA, Russell BD, Teram E, et al. Providing dental care to survivors of childhood sexual abuse: treatment considerations for the practitioner. J Am Dent Assoc 2005;136(9):1277–81.
21. Dougall A, Fiske J. Surviving child sexual abuse: the relevance to dental practice. Dent Update 2009;36:294–304.
22. Raja S, Hoersch M, Rajagopalan C, et al. Treating patients with traumatic life experiences. J Am Dent Assoc 2014;145(3):238–45.
23. Hamamoto DT, Rhodus NL. Methamphetamine abuse and dentistry. Oral Dis 2009;15:27–37.
24. Klasser GD, Epstein J. Methamphetamine and its impact on dental care. J Can Dent Assoc 2005;71(10):759–62.
25. Brodine AH, Hartshorn MA. Recognition and management of somatoform disorders. J Prosthet Dent 2004;91:268–73.
26. De Jongh A, Oosterink FMD, Aartman IHA. Preoccupation with one's appearance: a motivating factor for cosmetic dental treatment? Braz Dent J 2008; 204(12):691–5.
27. Friedlander AH, Serafetinides EA. Dental management of the patient with obsessive-compulsive disorder. Spec Care Dentist 1991;11(6):238–42.
28. Frydrych AM, Davies GR, McDermott BM. Eating disorders and oral health: a review of the literature. Aust Dent J 2005;50(1):6–15.
29. Clark DB. Patients with eating disorders: challenges for the oral health professional. Can J Dent Hyg 2010;44(4):163–70.

30. Lifant-Oliva C, Lopez-Jornet P, Camacho-Alonso F, et al. Study of oral changes in patients with eating disorders. Int J Dent Hyg 2008;6:119–22.
31. Liao CH, Chang CS, Muo CH, et al. High prevalence of herpes zoster in patients with depression. J Clin Psychiatry 2015;76(9):e1099–104.
32. Christensen L, Somers S. Comparison of nutrient intake among depressed and nondepressed individuals. Int J Eat Disord 1996;20(1):105–9.
33. Nierenberg AA, McIntyre RS, Sachs GS. Improving outcomes in patients with bipolar depression: a comprehensive review. J Clin Psychiatry Infopack 2015;2(2):1–12.
34. Rosmus L, Cobban SJ. Bipolar affective disorder and the dental hygienist. Can J Dent Hyg 2007;41(2):72–83.
35. Clark DB. Dental care for the patient with bipolar disorder. J Can Dent Assoc 2003;69(1):20–4.
36. Chuong R. Schizophrenia. Oral Surg Oral Med Oral Pathol Oral Radiol Endod 1999;88(5):526–8.
37. Friedlander A, Marder SR. The psychopathology, medical management and dental implications of schizophrenia. JADA 2002;133(5):603–10.
38. Clark DB. Dental care for the patient with schizophrenia. Can J Dent Hyg 2008;42(1):16–23.
39. Tenzer JA, Orozco H. Traumatic glossectomy. Oral Surg 1970;30:182–4.
40. MacLean G, Robertson BM. Self-enucleation and psychosis. Arch Gen Psychiatry 1976;33:242–9.
41. Mester R. The psychodynamics of the dental pathology of chronic schizophrenic patients. Isr J Psychiatry Relat Sci 1982;19:255–61.
42. Mitchell S. Advanced dementia. N Engl J Med 2015;372:2533–40.
43. Patil MS, Patil SB. Geriatric patient –psychological and emotional considerations during dental treatment. Gerodontology 2009;26:72–7.
44. Chalmers J, Johnson V. Evidence-based protocol. Oral hygiene care for functionally dependent and cognitively impaired older adults. J Gerontol Nurs 2004;11:5–12.
45. Hopcraft MS, Tan C. Xerostomia: an update for clinicians. Aust Dent J 2010;55:238–44.
46. Sonne SC, Brady KT. Bipolar disorder and alcoholism. Alcohol Res Health 2002;26(2):103–8. Available at: http://pubs.niaaa.nih.gov/publications/arh26-2/103-108.htm.
47. Ryan MCM, Thakore JH. Physical consequences of schizophrenia and its treatment. The metabolic syndrome. Life Sci 2002;71:239–57.
48. Parks J, Svendsen D, Singer P, et al, editors. Morbidity and mortality in people with serious mental illness. 2006. Available at: www.nasmhpd.org. Accessed October 6, 2015.
49. Goodell S, Druss BG, Walker ER. Mental disorders and medical comorbidity. Princeton, NJ: Robert Wood Johnson Foundation; 2011. Available at: http://www.rwjf.org/content/dam/farm/reports/issue_briefs/2011/rwjf69438.
50. Chapman DP, Perry GS, Strine TW. The vital link between chronic disease and depressive disorders. Prev Chronic Dis 2005;2(1):A14.
51. Cohn T. Schizophrenia and diabetes. Curr Psychiatry 2012;11(10):29–46.
52. Lunsky Y, Lin E, Balogh R, et al. Diabetes prevalence among persons with serious mental illness and developmental disability. Psychiatr Serv 2011;62(8):830.
53. Goldstein BI, Schaffer A, Wang S, et al. Excessive and premature new-onset cardiovascular disease among adults with bipolar disorder in the US NESARC Cohort. J Clin Psychiatry 2015;76(2):163–9.

54. Alberti KG, Zimmet P, Shaw J. Metabolic syndrome–a new world-wide definition. A consensus statement from the International Diabetes Federation. Diabet Med 2006;23(5):469–80.
55. Tremblay M, Gaudet D, Brison D. Metabolic syndrome and oral markers of cardiometabolic risk. J Can Dent Assoc 2011;77:b125. Available at: www.jcda.ca/article/b125.
56. Friedlander AH, Weintreb J, Friedlander I, et al. Metabolic syndrome: pathogenesis, medical care and dental implications. J Am Dent Assoc 2007;138(2): 179–87.
57. Mathus-Vliegen EM, Nikkel D, Brand HS. Oral aspects of obesity. Int Dent J 2007; 57(4):249–56.
58. Andriankaja OM, Sreenivasa S, Dunford R, et al. Association between metabolic syndrome and periodontal disease. Aust Dent J 2010;55:252–9.
59. Hennekens CH, Hennekens AR, Hollar D, et al. Schizophrenia and increased risks of cardiovascular disease. Am Heart J 2005;150:1115–21.
60. Lumby B. Guide schizophrenia patients to better physical health. Nurse Pract 2007;32(7):30–7.
61. Keene JJ, Galasko GT, Land MF. Antidepressant use in psychiatry and medicine. Importance for dental practice. JADA 2003;134(1):71–9.
62. Becker DE. Psychotropic drugs: implications for dental practice. Anesth Prog 2008;55:89–99.
63. Lieberman JA, Stroup TS, McEvoy JP, et al. Effectiveness of antipsychotic drugs in patients with chronic schizophrenia. N Engl J Med 2005;353(12):1209–23.
64. Gater L. Understanding xerostomia. AGD Impact 2006;34(6):6–8. Available at: http://www.agd.org/publications/articles/?artID=91.
65. Goldie MP. Xerostomia and quality of life. Int J Dent Hyg 2007;5:60–1.
66. Clark DB. Dental management considerations for patients with psychiatric disorders. Ont Dent 2006;83(1):22–5.
67. Swager LWM, Morgan SK. Psychotropic-induced dry mouth: don't overlook this potentially serious side effect. Curr Psychiatry 2011;10(12):54–8.
68. Oral health care for people with mental health problems. Guidelines and recommendations. 2000. Available at: http://www.bsdh.org.uk/guidelines-and-publications/Guidelines_Publications_Journals.php. Accessed October 6, 2015.
69. Blanchett PJ, Rompre PH, Lavigne GJ, et al. Oral dyskinesias: a clinical overview. Int J Prosthodont 2005;18:10–9.
70. Abidi S, Bhaskara SM. From chlorpromazine to clozapine–antipsychotic adverse effects and the clinician's dilemma. Can J Psychiatry 2003;48:749–55.
71. Sockalingham S, Shammi C, Remington G. Clozapine-induced hypersalivation: a review of treatment strategies. Can J Psychiatry 2007;52(6):377–84.
72. Wincour E, Gavish A, Voikovitch M, et al. Drugs and bruxism: a critical review. JOP 2003;17:99–111.
73. Brown ES, Hong SC. Antidepressant-induced bruxism successfully treated with gabapentin. JADA 1999;130:1467–9.
74. Ahmed KE. The psychology of tooth wear. Spec Care Dentist 2013;33(1):28–34.
75. De Hert M, Correll C, Cetovich-Bakmas M, et al. Physical illness in patients with severe mental disorders. I. Prevalence, impact of medications and disparities in health care. World Psychiatry 2011;10:52–77.
76. Comprehensive mental health action plan 2013-2020. Available at: http://www.who.int/mental_health/mhgap/consultation_global_mh_action_plan_2013_2020/en/index.html. Accessed October 15, 2015.

77. Kessler RC, Chiu WT, Demler O, et al. Prevalence, severity, and comorbidity of 12-month DSM-IV disorders in the National Comorbidity Survey Replication. Arch Gen Psychiatry 2005;62:617–27.
78. Godoy T, Riva A, Ekstrom J. Atypical antipsychotics–effects of amisulpride on salivary secretion and on clozapine-induced sialorrhea. Oral Dis 2012;18:680–91.

Tools and Equipment for Managing Special Care Patients Anywhere

Harvey Levy, DMD, MAGD, DABSCD[a,b], Lena R. Rotenberg, MS, MEd[a,]*

KEYWORDS

- Dental office • Equipment • Operating room • Portable dentistry
- Special care dentistry • Special needs patients • Tools • Hospital dentistry

KEY POINTS

- Successfully treating special care patients requires an investment in more than physical tools and equipment. Right personnel, right conversations with caregivers, right information, and right office layout are lynchpins to success.
- Most special care patients do not need to leave the security of their wheelchair, gurney, or bed for dental care, regardless of their medical or intellectual impairment. Many can come into your office or you can bring your portable equipment to them.
- It is fairly straightforward to provide excellent treatment to special care patients. Commercially available tools will allow you to gently immobilize and sedate these patients and to perform an oral examination, obtain a radiograph, and treat them in your office.
- In the minority of cases (for us, 4%) when office, homebound, or institutional treatment is not appropriate or possible, special care patients can be treated under general anesthesia in a hospital or surgical center operating room.

 Video content accompanies this article at http://www.dental.theclinics.com

INTRODUCTION

General dentists may be reluctant to accept special care patients into their practice because of negative beliefs so pervasive that we have identified and debunked 27 of them, referring to them as *myths*.[1] We have grouped the myths about treating

---

Disclosure Statement: The main author of this article has personally purchased and tested all the tools and equipment mentioned and chose to include specific brands and models based solely on their effectiveness in his practice. Some manufacturers (DentalEZ, Dental Film SRL, DEXIS, Isolite, KavoKerr Group, Porter Instrument, Septodont, Solutionreach, Specialized Care Inc, Ultralight Optics) will occasionally contribute toward his honoraria for courses and lectures at dental conferences. The coauthor has nothing to disclose.

[a] Dr. Harvey Levy & Associates, PC, 198 Thomas Johnson Drive, Suite 108, Frederick, MD 21702, USA; [b] Department of Surgery, Frederick Memorial Hospital, 400 W 7th Street, Frederick, MD 21701, USA
* Corresponding author.
E-mail address: drhlevy@gmail.com

special care patients into administrative barriers, management barriers, medical concerns, and financial concerns.

This article expands on specific management and medical myths, in particular, that

- It is difficult to work around these patients' wheelchairs and helmets.
- We dentists cannot do quality work because these patients do not cooperate.
- We are afraid of having to use oral sedation greater than the maximum recommended dose.
- We cannot obtain good radiographs.
- We are afraid of not being able to handle their emergencies.

With appropriate equipment and tools, and with the correct mindset by the dental team, treating special care patients presents only minor inconveniences as compared with treating everyone else.

Our practice in Frederick, Maryland has completed more than 36,000 special care patient visits over the past 42 years. This article addresses some tried and tested tools, techniques, and equipment that have allowed our doctors and staff to easily and effectively provide treatment to patients who require special attention.

In our case, they include patients who are autistic, medically compromised, intellectually disabled, uncooperative/combative, phobic, very young, or have Alzheimer's disease. We see such patients in assisted-living facilities, in nursing homes and other institutions, in private homes, in hospices, and bedside at the hospital. We treat a small percentage of these patients in the hospital or surgical center operating room.

Because of the clinically pragmatic nature of this article and because so much of it is based on our own experience, we mostly use first person and address the reader as *you*. We hope you are comfortable with that.

We have adopted a broad definition of *tool* to encompass 3-dimensional spaces and objects as well as conceptual tools. Concrete tools include the physical setup of the office space in addition to tried and tested equipment commercially available for purchase that will enable you to successfully treat patients with special needs inside and outside your office. Conceptual tools include clinical and behavioral techniques and procedures we use with our patients, which must necessarily go beyond the usual please-open-your-mouth directive.

Our basis for selecting one tool over another is how well it works in our practice with its more than 2,000 active special care patients treated in a wide variety of settings.

This article is organized sequentially, from pretreatment to treatment. Thus, we will begin with the most important element we bring to the treatment of special care patients: the clinician's attitude. Without the right personnel, any tool loses effectiveness.

BEFORE YOU BEGIN
Having the Right Personnel

All the tools and equipment in the world will not make you successful treating special care patients unless *everyone* in your practice welcomes them in wholeheartedly. Patients can sense an unsafe environment, a negative or fearful attitude, or trepidation emanating from your staff. If you are committed to treating special care patients, you will lead by example and you will attract a dental team who shares your caring attitude toward these patients and their caregivers, welcoming them into your practice.

The number of dental staff in the treatment room, whether for a doctor or hygiene visit, will depend on the individual patient and the caregivers who accompany them. The number is typically 3. If 6 or more people are needed to calm and restrain a patient, we take the patient to a hospital or surgical center operating room (OR) and treat them under general anesthesia.

To establish rapport in the treatment room, it is best if clinicians position themselves at the patient's eye level or lower, place their hand on the patient's hand or shoulder, and make eye contact from below to reduce the white coat intimidation factor.

Having the Right Conversations: Getting Information About Your Special Care Patients

Special care patients are as unique as fingerprints and snowflakes. If you have treated one autistic patient, you have treated one autistic patient; the next one you treat will respond differently. The initial conversation with a patient's caregivers when the appointment is made will enable you to become aware of what works for that patient. You may also have to contact their former dentists and physicians to learn what treatments were performed, how the patient responded, and what they learned about the patient.

Next are some questions that we typically ask caregivers and former doctors of special care patients, in addition to the standard questions we ask every patient.

- What techniques and drugs were tried previously? What succeeded and what failed?
- What are the patient's likes and dislikes (fears and phobias) in a clinical setting?
- Does the patient like any special music that we can play in the treatment room?
- Who assists the patient with their oral hygiene, and what methods are used?
- What are the patient's negative triggers, such as bright lights, loud noises, touching, too many people in the room?
- What would the patient consider to be a threatening environment?
- Are there any medical or health problems we need to be aware of?

The last and most important question we ask is always, what else do YOU think we should know?

Having the Right Information

Most of our special care patients are on multiple drugs. The most effective means we found to prevent a synergistic or antagonistic response with further drugs we prescribe is Lexicomp Online. We simply type in the drugs the patients are taking, add the drugs we are considering, and check for adverse effects. This necessary precaution helps us follow our Hippocratic mandate to *above all, do no harm*.

Having the Right Office Layout

The architecture of your office building and how your rooms are set up will determine which special care patients you will be able to treat in-house. In the past 25 years the Americans with Disabilities Act[2] codes have mandated improvements that have made most office buildings accessible, so we will not talk about external doors, parking spaces, ramps, stairs, and elevators.

Next are some characteristics of our physical layout and procedures we follow to reduce physical barriers to care at our office.

- Versatility: All our treatment rooms are set up lefty/righty convertible. Patients can enter most treatment rooms from either side. Much of our operatory furniture is movable and removable. The x-ray units are fixed to the walls, but we have access to handheld units as well.

- Psychological barriers: On request of a caregiver, we may prescribe sedative drugs for patients reluctant to come into our office. We may also provide photographs or a video of what the patients' path to our treatment room will look like, so that they can be coached in advance of their first visit.
- Communication: We urge caregivers to call us from their vehicle if patients need assistance entering our building or getting into our office.
- Equipment to aid mobility: We are able to provide a wheelchair, a walker, and mobility/sliding boards to patients who are unable or unwilling to walk into our office.
- Waiting room: Our waiting room has a designated area for patients on a wheelchair, and there is a clear path for easy entry and exit of a wheelchair or gurney.
- Reception windows and counters: Our reception windows and counters are low enough to enable eye contact between patients and our front desk staff. We have installed bilevel countertops whereby the lower level is used by patients in wheelchairs to conduct normal business with the front desk staff (**Fig. 1**).
- Oversize bathroom with hand railing: We require all nondiapered patients taking any sedation drugs or laughing gas to empty their bladder immediately before entering the treatment room. Our facilities accommodate wheelchairs and patients with walkers.[3]
- Path to treatment rooms: Our corridors are straight and wide enough to enable large motorized wheelchairs and long gurneys to reach the treatment rooms (Video 1). We have tested our pathways to ensure that wheelchairs and gurneys are able to negotiate all the turns necessary to enter and depart all our treatment rooms.

SEATING PATIENTS
Movable Operatory Chairs

If your chair is attached to the floor, it may be difficult for you and your staff to develop an excellent traffic pattern around your treatment room. Some patients may approach

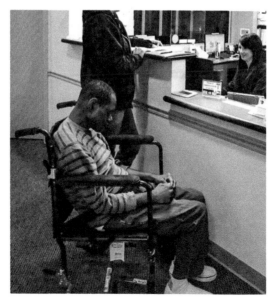

Fig. 1. Bilevel countertop.

your chair from behind a cane or a walker or from a wheelchair, requiring additional space to enter and exit your chair. Be careful with hoses, foot controls, operatory lights, and bracket tables that may be obstacles.[4]

Some special care patients are downright unable or unwilling to move from their gurney or wheelchair into our operatory chair. Patients with Alzheimer's disease often do not like to be moved; autistic patients usually do not like to be touched; obese patients and amputees cannot readily be moved. Movable operatory chairs, which we move off to the side in a couple of seconds, enable us to treat these patients in the security of their own familiar chariot placed in the center of our treatment room (**Fig. 2**).

In our 9 treatment rooms we use the DentalEZ J-Chair (DentalEZ, Bay Minette, AL) equipped with the optional Air Glide base (**Fig. 3**A, B). At the push of a button, activated with a finger or toe, a diaphragm at the base of the chair is inflated and even a small child is able to move the hovercraft-style chair in any direction (Video 2). As an added bonus, we often allow small children to become comfortable in our treatment room by giving them a free ride while they sit in the chair. The size and cost of these chairs is equivalent to those of most standard chairs. A newer model is the Nu-Simplicity chair.

Seating children or small-statured adult patients in these chairs is discussed later (see Seating and Restraining Short-Statured Patients), together with applying physical restraints for their protection.

Supporting Patients' Heads on Their Own Wheelchairs

Special care patients who come in wearing a helmet are predisposed to self-injury. They are likely to jerk their heads into a needle, drill, probe, or other sharp tool and

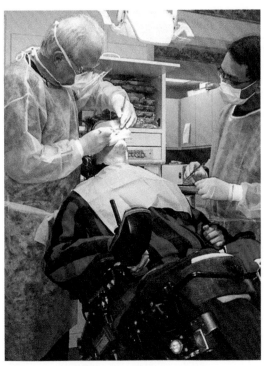

Fig. 2. Patient receiving care in own wheelchair.

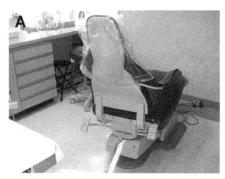
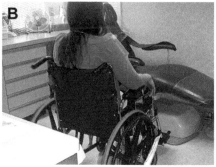

Fig. 3. Movable chair makes room for a wheelchair. (*A*) Treatment room with DentalEZ chair in the center. (*B*) Treatment room with DentalEZ chair moved aside. (*Courtesy of* DentalEZ, Bay Minette, AL; with permission.)

require special attention. We remove the helmet when the head can be safely immobilized and protected by pillows, Velcro (Velcro Inc, Manchester, NH), straps, or a caregiver's hands.

We may use a removable commercial headrest, clipped onto the patient's own wheelchair.[5] Alternatively, we may clip a removable headrest onto our own operatory chair facing backwards and align the operatory chair back-to-back with the patient's wheelchair, so that the head of the patient rests on the operatory chair's reverse headrest. The most effective headrest is the chest of a caregiver or staff member. That person's hands and chest provide excellent head immobility, coupled with often-needed versatility (**Fig. 4**).

Transferring Patients from Wheelchair to Operatory Chair

Patients or caregivers will usually bring their own mobility or sliding boards to enable transfer back and forth from car seat to a wheelchair and from wheelchair to your operatory chair (**Fig. 5**). Patients and caregivers have their preferred transfer methods and most often will not require your help.[6]

Mobility/sliding boards: Straight and arched beveled wooden boards allow patients to slide from one chair to another, with or without assistance.[5] A variety of such commercial boards is available.

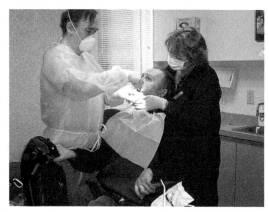

Fig. 4. Dental assistant positioned to also serve as headrest.

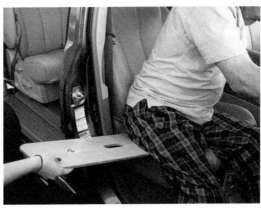

Fig. 5. Patient transfers from vehicle to wheelchair (and after that to operatory chair) via wooden sliding board.

Carrying patients: When patients do require assistance, our staff members are proficient in the 2-person transfer method.[7,8] Staff are also able to perform the one-person transfer, which relies on pivoting the patient on their own feet.[5]

IMMOBILIZING PATIENTS

When patients are unable or unwilling to comply with our requests to sit still, open their mouth, or turn their head, we can use chemical and/or physical restraints to ensure their compliance and immobility so that we can do our best work without anyone getting injured. These two modalities for immobilizing patients are synergistic.

Chemical Restraints

A growing trend in special care dentistry is intravenous (IV) sedation,[9] which we currently choose not to use in our office. IV sedation requires a patient recovery room, a designated area with a couch, emergency equipment, and suction equipment that must be approved by a site visit team.[10] Many dentists choose to bring in an anesthesiologist or a nurse anesthetist instead of undergoing the additional academic and clinical training required to obtain a permit. Staff must also be trained in these circumstances. Although IV sedation is generally considered safe, complications may arise.[11]

The chemical restraints that we use to treat special care patients in our office encompass mild to moderate oral conscious sedation and nitrous oxide (laughing gas). Patients we take to the OR receive general anesthesia.

Oral conscious sedation

We have had most success with the benzodiazepine sedatives, which include either liquid or pill diazepam (Valium), triazolam (Halcion), and lorazepam (Ativan). We also occasionally use other sedatives/hypnotics. We use such chemical restraints across all ages and weight ranges, with special attention to their lowest effective doses and maximum recommended doses as listed in the *Physicians Desk Reference*.

Patients are asked to come to the office on a 6-hour empty stomach in order to prevent aspiration during the visit. We ask caregivers to give patients any oral sedatives 30 minutes before the scheduled appointment time (nothing by mouth). We want the medicine to peak when we are in the mouth and not when patients first arrive to do chart updates and go to the bathroom to empty their bladder.

Nitrous oxide/laughing gas

Nitrous oxide is considered the safest sedative available, with no contraindications as long as an adequate percentage of oxygen is administered[12] and standard procedures and cautions are followed.[13] We use nitrous oxide to increase patients' pain threshold and to keep them relaxed, sedated, and often amnesic. Patients must be on an empty bladder and stomach, except for prescribed medicine.

In all our treatment rooms we have installed the built-in Porter Nitrous Oxide Sedation System. We also have one of their portable units, which we use occasionally when patients need oxygen in the waiting room. The built-in system is designed to shut off automatically if the proportion of oxygen decreases to less than 30%.

We now use their Silhouette disposable nitrous oxide nasal mask, whose lower profile is less obtrusive and more acceptable to patients than older models (**Fig. 6**). These masks do not interfere with patients' safety glasses or sunglasses, a capability especially appreciated by photophobic autistic patients for whom most lights are a negative trigger.

To help patients accept the nitrous oxide mask, we ask them their favorite fruit or flavor. We use that flavor of Lip Smacker to coat the lining of their mask. We also write the patient's name on the mask and at the end of the visit give them the mask to take home as a reward for good behavior.

When patients receive nitrous oxide without any other sedation medicine, they may drive themselves home or back to work with no impairment or residual sedative side effects. The drug's sedative and anxiolytic effects are gone only minutes after turning off and removing the nitrous oxide mask.

Conscious sedation plus nitrous oxide

We use a blood pressure cuff and pulse oximeter on patients who receive either oral conscious sedation and nitrous oxide (**Fig. 7**). Requirements vary from state to state whether such monitoring is required or optional. When nitrous oxide is used in conjunction with oral conscious sedation, our rate of success in completing treatment is significantly higher than either one alone.

Physical Restraints

Recently there has been an outcry against physically restraining dental patients, particularly small children and mentally compromised adults. Physical restraint has been deemed "shameful" and "inhumane," especially the hand-over-mouth-exercise technique or application of a wrestling style "headlock."[14] A more measured approach

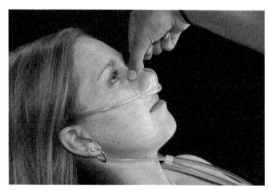

Fig. 6. Patient relaxing with Silhouette nitrous oxide mask. (*Courtesy of* Parker Hannifin Corporation, Porter Instrument Division, Hatfield, PA; with permission.)

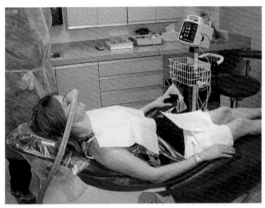

Fig. 7. Patient wearing nitrous mask monitored by blood pressure cuff and pulse oximeter.

deems physical restraints acceptable and states that there are some areas of agreement regarding their use:

- It should only be used when necessary.
- The least restrictive alternative should be used.[15]
- Restraint shall not be used as punishment or for the convenience of staff.
- Restraints should cause no physical injury to patients.[16]

A comprehensive review of protective stabilization equipment for pediatric dental patients adds other considerations, such as its ability to be disinfected and appropriately sized.[17]

The wood-based Papoose Board, with its rigid back that does not contour to the operatory chair, has been judged acceptable by mothers who witnessed its use with their own small children[18] but unacceptable when presented via a videotape of what might happen.[19] Ultimately, the legal guardians of special care patients must balance many factors, including the higher cost and medical risk of deep IV sedation or general anesthesia, as they provide their informed consent to different patient behavior management techniques.

In our treatment rooms we offer gentle physical restraints with body wraps made of soft breathable mesh fabric and Velcro, most often used in conjunction with oral sedation and/or nitrous oxide.

Body wraps

We use the Rainbow Wraps by Specialized Care Co. These body wraps, made of colorful breathable mesh and Velcro, come in 6 sizes and restrict patients' entire body from the neck to the knees. They are nonthreatening, breathable, comfortable, easy to apply, and contour to the operatory chair (**Figs. 8–10**).

Rainbow Wraps may either contain a split on the side to allow a pulse oximeter on a finger (stock item), or wrap the whole body to prevent a hand from escaping out (Carolyn Fetter, personal communication, 2015). Both models include 2 Velcro wristbands to reduce movement (**Fig. 9**).

The Specialized Care Co also sells the Knee Belt, a separate wrap for the knees and/or ankles, which is merely a long strip of Velcro. Should there be the slightest likelihood that patients will kick a clinician, we use the knee belt in addition to the Rainbow Wrap to restrain the feet (**Fig. 8**).

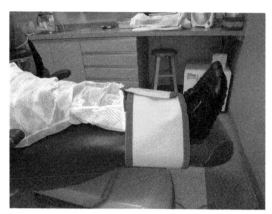

Fig. 8. Rainbow Wrap's Knee Belt is placed around the knees and/or ankles to prevent kicking. (*Courtesy of* specialized Care Co Inc, Hampton, NH; with permission.)

We also may use a narrower strip of Velcro to secure the patient's head to our headrest or to the headrest mounted on their own wheelchair. The Specialized Care Co calls it a Head Strap.

Seating and restraining short-statured patients
For young patients, an extremely effective way to seat them is on their caregiver's lap. The caregiver sits on the dental chair, and holds the body-wrapped child on their lap. The additional benefit of contact between the caregiver and child during treatment, which we always encourage, is welcomed by mothers of young children (**Fig. 10**).[18]

In lieu of a caregiver, we use the Stay N Place Chair Cushion by Specialized Care Co, a chair insert that looks and feels like a mini foam mattress and inserts completely and comfortably onto any of our DentalEZ operatory chairs (**Fig. 11**).

Restraining by touching
One of the most effective means to restrain special care patients is to touch them, which reassures them that their caregiver is present and protecting them. After

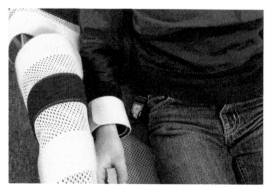

Fig. 9. Wrists wrapped inside Rainbow Wrap to reduce movement. (*Courtesy of* Specialized Care Co Inc, Hampton, NH; with permission.)

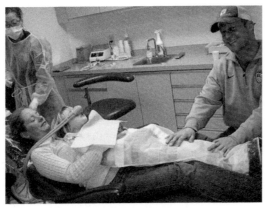

Fig. 10. Sedated, wrapped child on mother's lap with nitrous mask and father's supportive touch.

patients are wrapped in a Rainbow Wrap, there are 3 levels of touch that we may ask caregivers to provide during treatment.

- Finger: The caregiver places a finger or hand on the patient's arms or torso.
- Two hands on two hands: The caregiver presses down on the patient's wrists, discouraging any attempt to break out.
- Straddle: The caregiver straddles the patient's legs with their own feet still on the floor, facing the patient. This placement prevents any sudden movements of the patient's torso.

Psychological Techniques

Special care patients amenable to a caregiver restraining them with touch have the added benefit of seeing a known face and hearing a known voice in the operatory, which contributes to their feeling safe and not threatened or abandoned.

Patients with autism spectrum disorder, however, seldom like to be touched. Furthermore, they rarely follow the normal algorithms of behavior modification or titration effect; more often than not, increased sedation has a reverse or paradoxical effect.

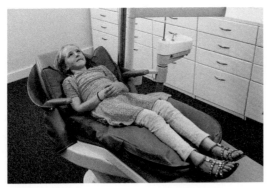

Fig. 11. A portable Stay N Place Chair Cushion converts an adult operatory chair into children's size. (*Courtesy of* specialized Care Co Inc, Hampton, NH; with permission.)

Many autistic patients have triggers that we can avoid (**Fig. 12**A, B):

- Not liking to be touched: If we do not have time for long-term desensitization therapy, we decrease their sensitivity to touch by using laughing gas and/or sedative drugs.
- Photophobic: We give them opaque sunglasses or blackout eye shades; the doctor wears a headlight that focuses light directly in the mouth, such as the Feather Light LED mentioned later.
- Noise: If the drill and dental office sounds irritate them, we give them ear plugs or sound-reducing headphones, which may or may not be connected to a soothing sound source.
- Smells: To those offended by normal dental smells, we offer nose plugs.

Our best practice is to ask the caregiver what helps to set the patient at ease and what triggers we should address. Quite often caregivers will bring headphones and an electronic tablet loaded with whatever media best soothes and calms the patient. Otherwise, we offer mental age-appropriate videos and television channels, usually helpful to distract patients.

PATIENTS WHO CANNOT COME TO YOUR OFFICE

Sometimes special care patients cannot come to the dental office, and you will be asked to visit them in

- Private homes (patients hooked up to machines, morbidly obese, leg amputees, agoraphobic, Alzheimer's autistic)
- Nursing homes (patients whose health or mental status precludes them from being brought to the office)

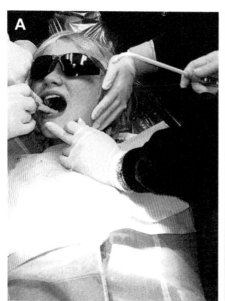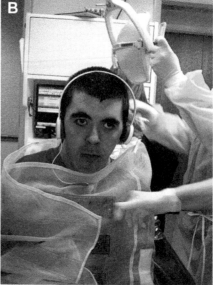

Fig. 12. Avoiding common triggers of autistic patients. (*A*) Opaque sunglasses on photophobic patient. (*B*) Sound-reducing headphones worn by acousticophobic patient.

- Institutions or hospital bedside (patients with psychological illness, patients with an infectious disease who cannot leave their wards, or patients in the intensive care unit)
- Hospice (patients too frail to leave the building)

At such locations, we may not need to physically wrap patients, but they may be sedated and/or restrained by family or staff present.

We are successful in the dental office and in the field treating 96% of our special care patients. The remaining 4% are uncooperative and cannot be diagnosed, or their treatments require lighting and suction beyond what is available outside the dental office, or require treatment too extensive for us to administer without general anesthesia. In such cases we bring patients to the OR.[20]

The tools and equipment we describe in subsequent sections can be used in your operatory or in the field. Tools that we also bring to the OR are explicitly indicated. The only piece of equipment that we use in the OR and nowhere else is a throat pack to close the airway and to prevent any water, chemicals, or objects from being aspirated into the lungs (**Fig. 13**).

The supplies, tools, and equipment we use in the OR are the same as in the office, with patients asleep on an OR table instead of consciously sedated in a dental chair.

DIAGNOSTIC PHASE

Once special care patients are seated, immobilized, and sedated, we follow the normal diagnostic steps as for any other patient:

- Oral examination including periodontal evaluation to whatever extent is possible, cancer screening, and check for caries, fractures, abscesses, and other pathologic conditions
- Radiographs
- Photographs and/or intraoral video
- Treatment plan

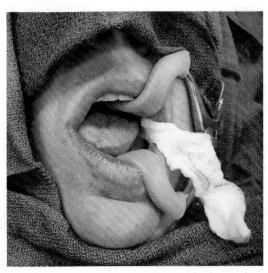

Fig. 13. Throat pack and Molt mouth gag on patient under hospital general anesthesia.

Oral Examination

We use the tools and procedures discussed next to perform oral examinations on special care patients both in our office or when seeing them outside our office.

Opening the mouth

Most of our special care patients do not comply when we request that they open the mouth. We have adopted several acupressure techniques (using acupuncture points) that enable us to get a patient to open fairly quickly, using a simple momentary distraction. Our success rate in thousands of attempts is 98%.

Our favorite technique is vibrating the chin button at the bottom of the mentolabial groove directly below the lower lip (conception point 24[21]). Apply vibrating pressure at a 45° angle downward with your finger or knuckle while supporting the forehead (Video 3). We may also pinch the nose just long enough for patients to open the mouth, allowing us to insert a mouth prop (**Fig. 14**A, B).

Other pressure-point mouth-opening techniques are beyond the scope of this article but are taught in our participation courses.[22]

Keeping the mouth open

Once we get a patient's mouth open, we need to keep it open. Our best results are obtained by horizontally inserting a soft Open Wide Mouth Rest, a wooden tongue depressor surrounded by white foam made by the Specialized Care Co, then rotating it 90°.

We then insert a Molt mouth gag on the opposite side, which allows us to gently ratchet the mouth open as wide as necessary to complete the task (**Fig. 15**). Once the Molt gag is in, we remove the mouth rest.

After slowly opening the mouth to the maximum with Molt gag, we keep one finger on its hinge at all times. That prevents the patient's tongue from dislodging the gag and potentially clamping down on the sharp object in their mouth or on your finger.

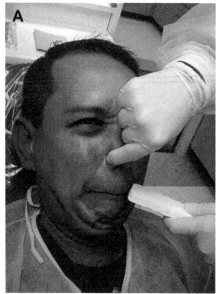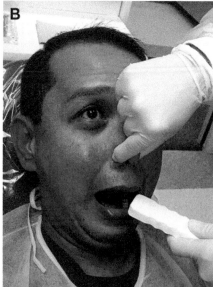

Fig. 14. Technique to encourage the patient to open the mouth. (*A*) Pinch the nose. (*B*) Insert foam mouth rest when patient opens momentarily.

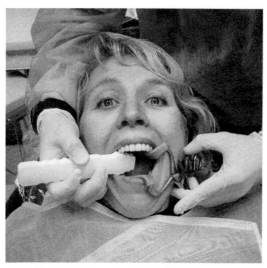

Fig. 15. Inserting and ratcheting Molt mouth gag before removing foam mouth rest.

When ready to switch sides, we insert a second Molt mouth gag before withdrawing the first. If you do not have a second Molt gag, then close the ratchet and rotate it 180° as you move to the other side without withdrawing the gag. Then, slowly expand it to maximum opening and place a finger on the hinge.

Another tool we use to prop the mouth open is the bilateral Jennings mouth prop,[23] found in ears, nose, and throat catalogues (**Fig. 16**). This gag is indicated when working on the 12 anterior teeth, as it opens the mouth at the premolars. We also use a wide variety of standard unilateral rubber or plastic props known to most dentists.

Illumination
Whenever special care patients keep moving their heads out of the beam of the operatory overhead light, we wear a battery-operated, rechargeable, Ultralight Optics headlight, the Feather Light LED. This featherweight loupe-light can be hooked on

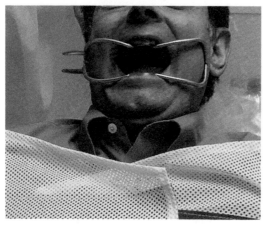

Fig. 16. Bilateral Jennings mouth prop.

to either prescription glasses or safety glasses and used in conjunction with loops if desired. The clinician is able to keep the work field lit by merely following the patient's head movements (**Fig. 17**). This headlight is especially useful to treat autistic photophobic patients or to perform a hands-free examination and treatment off-site.

Oral cancer screening device

Whenever we conduct an intraoral examination of patients in our office, in a hospital, private home, nursing home, hospice center, or even sitting on the floor (some patients refuse to sit on a waiting room chair), we use the wandlike Identafi Oral Cancer Screening System. Its internal light powerfully illuminates the mouth while retracting the patient's cheeks and frees up our other hand to hold an explorer, probe, or scaler (**Fig. 18**).

By shining different frequencies of light on the soft tissue, abnormalities are more easily detected (**Fig. 19**).[24] We also check for enamel crazes in anterior teeth. In the past 2 years we have successfully identified 2 new squamous cell carcinomas with the aid of this device.

Checking for caries

If for whatever reason we cannot get a radiograph for a patient, we use the DEXIS CariVu to check for carious lesions and cracks. This novel device, which looks like a small flashlight, uses a safe, near-infrared light to scan the teeth and display carious lesions as dark areas (**Fig. 20**). This tool is very well received by most of our special care patients. It is also useful when any patient does not consent to having radiographs taken.

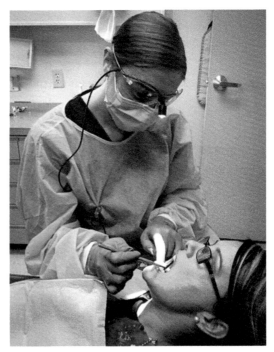

Fig. 17. Ultralight optics headlight. (*Courtesy of* Ultralight Optics, Costa Mesa, CA; with permission.)

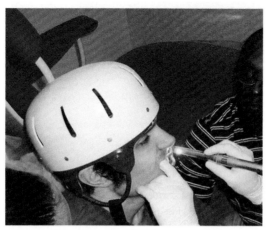

Fig. 18. Identafi used to examine a patient on the floor. (*Courtesy of* DentalEZ, Bay Minette, AL; with permission.)

Radiographs

An x-ray system is to a dentist like a stethoscope is to a cardiologist; we go in without these tools at the risk of incomplete or improper diagnosis. The tools and equipment discussed later help us obtain excellent or reasonable radiographs on special care patients anywhere.

Handheld x-ray unit

In our office treatment rooms we use the standard wall-mounted x-ray units. In the hospital OR we bring in one of their x-ray units on wheels. Neither of those x-ray units is portable, a feature necessary to diagnose special care patients wherever they may be.

The cordless rechargeable battery operated NOMAD Pro and NOMAD Pro 2 handheld x-ray systems by Aribex weigh approximately 5.5 lb. They enable us to safely take radiographs bedside in hospitals, nursing homes, private homes, hospice centers, and institutions and to conduct public dental screenings. These units are also used as our primary backup in the office, hospital, and surgical center.

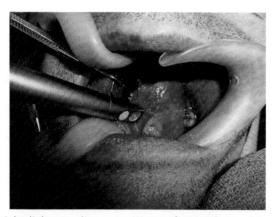

Fig. 19. Identafi violet light revealing a suspicious soft tissue lesion. (*Courtesy of* DentalEZ, Bay Minette, AL; with permission.)

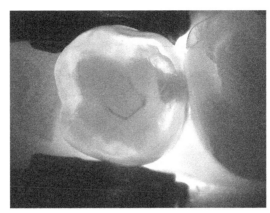

Fig. 20. CariVu (DEXIS, Hatfield, PA) image of molar caries. (*Courtesy of* DEXIS, Hatfield, PA, with permission.)

An apron-protected assistant exposing a digital sensor with this handheld unit can see instantly if the exposure time needs to be adjusted or if the radiograph needs to be retaken for any other reason. There is no walking or waiting. We can obtain safe and accurate radiographs quickly, an important benefit with patients who often do not give us a large working window.

Digital x-ray and imaging system
For many years we have used the DEXIS digital sensor (both the classic and the Platinum types) together with the DEXIS dental software, which integrates with Dentrix, our patient management software. We also use the DEXshield, a radiation-shielding positioning ring.

With this system our assistants or hygienists can take a full series of 18 radiographs in 5 minutes, resulting in clear and detailed images obtained with a low dose of radiation. The DEXIS sensor connects via USB to our operatory desktop computer or to a laptop on which the DEXIS software was installed.

We bring our DEXIS x-ray system with us when seeing patients at any location, including the OR. As long as the batteries are charged on both the handheld x-ray unit and on the laptop to which the DEXIS sensor is connected, we are able to capture excellent quality radiographs literally anywhere (**Fig. 21**A–D).

X-ray film
In the absence of DEXIS digital capabilities, we use the analog D-Speed Ergonom-X Dental Film (self-developing film) by Dental Film SRL as our backup. This inexpensive self-contained size 2 film manufactured in Italy and widely available in the United States is enclosed in a packet with its own chemical fixer and developer. There is no metal in the packet to create a herringbone artifact. This film is commonly used as a primary dental imaging system in off-site locations, such as overseas missions and field hospitals (**Fig. 22**A–C).

After exposing an image as one would with any size 2 film, it is processed and developed in 60 seconds by merely massaging the film packet with one's fingers (see YouTube video[25]). The images are quite good and may be scanned for archival purposes. No computers, electricity, darkroom, or loose chemicals are needed.

Panoramic imaging
Many of our special care patients will not tolerate intraoral radiographs. The Planmeca ProMax 2D S2 panoramic imaging unit that we use is versatile enough to allow

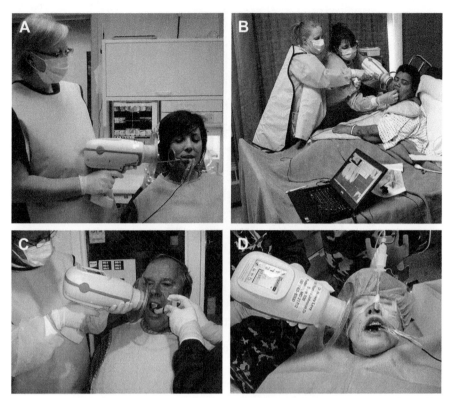

Fig. 21. NOMAD-Pro with DEXIS sensor capturing images in various locations. (*A*) In office operatory. (*B*) In nursing home or hospice on nonambulatory patient. (*C*) In waiting room. (*D*) In OR. ([*A*] *Courtesy of* KaVo Kerr Group, Wood Dale, IL; with permission; [*B*] *Courtesy of* DEXIS, Hatfield, PA, with permission.)

wheelchair access and can take extraoral bitewings in addition to panoramic images (**Fig. 23**).

We drape a lead-free panoramic poncho by Dux Dental around patients as well as the caregiver and/or assistant as needed to obtain one or 2 images. Often imperfections on the first image do not coincide with imperfections on the second, and with 2 images we may have enough diagnostic data to formulate a tentative treatment plan.

Photographs and Intraoral Video

We use a DEXcam 3 intraoral camera to take intraoral photographs and video of patients, with signed consent from caregivers, to serve as a backup to radiographs and also as additional input to develop a treatment plan, confer with colleagues, or preauthorize with a dental insurance carrier. We shoot video when special care patients move too quickly for us to take still shots, filming at various angles and directions (**Fig. 24**). We are later able to select specific images from the tongue's perspective in order to diagnose and develop a treatment plan.

Treatment Plan

Armed with data collected from the oral examination, radiographs, and photographs, we prepare one or more treatment plans that we submit to the legal guardian for

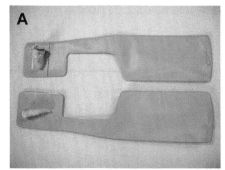
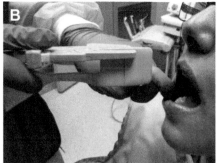
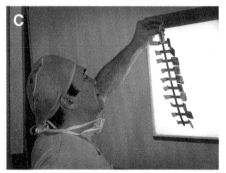

Fig. 22. Ergonom-X dental film. (*A*) Extracted teeth placed on dental film. (*B*) Placement of dental film. (*C*) Self-developing film drying on a hanger in the OR. (*Courtesy of* Dental Film SRL, Settimo Torinese, TO, Italy; with permission.)

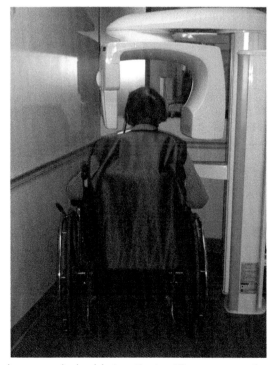

Fig. 23. DUX Poncho-aproned wheelchair patient getting a panoramic radiograph and extraoral bitewings. (*Courtesy of* DUX Dental, Oxnard, CA; with permission.)

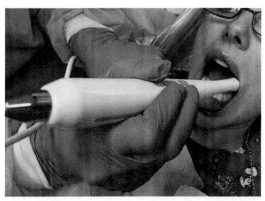

Fig. 24. DEXcam capturing multiple images in patient's mouth. (*Courtesy of* DEXIS, Hatfield, PA; with permission.)

selection, approval, and consent. Depending on the complexity of the treatment and the patient's comfort level in our office, we choose whether to treat in the office or the OR and decide whether treatment will be performed in one or multiple visits.

TREATMENT
Dental Isolation Devices

We have great success with the Isolite series of mouth props, which come in various sizes. The clear plastic props include a tongue retractor, cheek retractor, saliva ejector, high-volume evacuator, and 3 levels of intraoral light (**Fig. 25**).

This soft, comfortable, and helpful 5-in-1 device was designed for application of sealants, composites, and other restorations. It keeps the mouth open while drying, isolating, and illuminating the area.

Portable and Mobile Carts

A mobile cart can be wheeled from one area to another, for example, in a hospital. A portable cart can fit into the trunk of a vehicle and transported to an off-site location (**Fig. 26**). We have used various carts by DNTLworks and Aseptico mobile units and

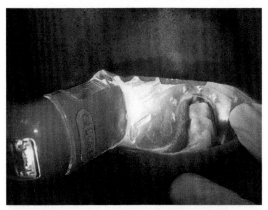

Fig. 25. The clear plastic props include a tongue retractor, cheek retractor, throat obturation, dual quadrant evacuation, 5-levels of intraoral light. (*Courtesy of* Isolite Systems, Santa Barbara, CA; with permission.)

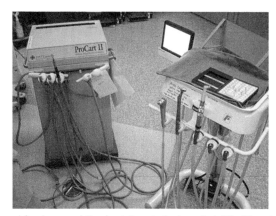

Fig. 26. Primary and backup mobile dental carts in hospital OR. (*Courtesy of* DNTLworks Equipment Corporation, Centennial, CO, with permission; and Aseptico, Inc, Woodinville, WA, with permission.)

have found them to be quite powerful, especially when used in conjunction with the Feather Light LED lights discussed earlier.

EMERGENCY MEDICAL SUPPLIES AND EQUIPMENT
Medical Emergency Kit

We compiled our own emergency kit, which includes an automatic external defibrillator (AED), and keep it close to our operatories (**Fig. 27**). Commercial kits (eg, Zoll or HealthFirst) include perishable/disposable goods (gloves, thermometers, gauze, epinephrine injection [EpiPen], needles, alcohol, plastic airway, sugar, drugs) and durable equipment (thermometer, blood pressure cuff, tourniquet, syringes), with which we stock our own kit. Twice a year we hold an office-wide emergency drill whereby we rehearse AED use and the ABCs of cardiopulmonary resuscitation.

Essential Drugs

In our medical emergency kit we always carry 2 essential drugs in addition to the standard drugs required for our Moderate Sedation permit.

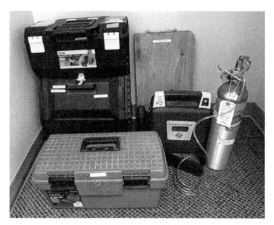

Fig. 27. Medical emergency equipment always available.

Phentolamine mesylate (OraVerse): At the end of a case we may inject this drug into the same site as the local anesthetic agent in order to reverse the lip, tongue, or cheek numbing effect of our local anesthetics,[26] especially when special care patients are prone to bite their own lip, tongue, or cheek (**Fig. 28**).

Flumazenil (Romazicon)[27]: Flumazenil is the only effective reversal agent available to counter the benzodiazepines we administer to our special care patients. To date we have never had to use it, but we often rehearse how to inject this life-saving drug in the event of accidental overdose or unexpected respiratory depression from the Valium, Halcion, or Ativan we prescribe. If we cannot get the reversal drug quickly into a vein, we are prepared to inject it under the highly vascular tongue intraorally or, if necessary, extraorally from under the chin.

SUMMARY

In 2010 nearly 20% of the American population had a severe disability.[28] We have offered effective solutions in the form of tools and equipment that, in our experience, disclaim widespread myths about treating special care patients. It is not difficult to work around patients' wheelchairs or deal with their helmets. Chemical and physical restraints enable dentists to do excellent-quality work; if they fail, we can bring patients to the OR and provide care under general anesthesia.[29] Reasonably good radiographs can be taken literally anywhere, even when there is no electricity. Finally, special care patients' emergencies are even less likely than other patients' if their recent and accurate health history is available.

The tools and equipment described in this article can be viewed at dental meetings, dental supply showrooms, courses, or during in-office lunch-and-learn

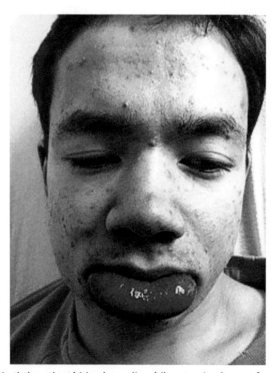

Fig. 28. Effect of Autistic patient biting lower lip while returning home after dental treatment.

demonstrations. If you are committed to providing a high standard of care to under-served special care patient populations, we urge you to explore and experiment to find out which tools work best for you.

SUPPLEMENTARY DATA

Supplementary data related to this article can be found at http://dx.doi.org/10.1016/j. cden.2016.03.001.

REFERENCES

1. Levy H. Debunking the myths about special-needs patient care. Dentaltown Magazine 2010;11(8):62–5. Available at: http://www.dentaltown.com/dentaltown/article. aspx?aid=2842. Accessed November 5, 2015.
2. Americans with Disabilities Act of 1990, as amended in 2008, 42 USC §§12101 et seq. Available at: http://www.ada.gov/pubs/adastatute08.htm. Accessed November 5, 2015.
3. United States Access Board. A guide to ADAAG provisions. Available at: http://www.access-board.gov/guidelines-and-standards/buildings-and-sites/113-ada-standards/background/adaag/422-a-guide-to-adaag-provisions#Toilet. Accessed November 5, 2015.
4. Suarez P. Wheelchair transfers, presentation. Herman Ostrow School of Dentistry of University of Southern California. January 29, 2009. Available at: http://www.usc.edu/hsc/dental/GSPD504/WT.pdf. Accessed November 1, 2015.
5. Jolly DE. Wheelchair transfer. Presentation. "Wheelchair headrest in use" slide. Available at: http://www.wheelchairnet.org/wcn_living/Docs/DisabilityWheelchair.pdf. Accessed November 1, 2015.
6. Timby BK. Assisting with basic needs. Fundamentals of nursing skills and concepts. In: Timby BK, editor. Fundamentals of nursing skills and concepts. 9th edition. Philadelphia: Lippincott Williams & Wilkins; 2008. p. 528.
7. U.S. Department of Health and Human Services. Wheelchair transfer: a health provider guide. 2004. Publication No. 04-5195. Available at: http://dhonline.chattanoogastate.edu/modules/specialneeds/Mabe/2015%20Special%20needs/Disability/wheelchair%20handout.pdf. Accessed November 1, 2015.
8. Suarez P. Wheelchair transfers, presentation. 2009. Available at: http://www.usc.edu/hsc/dental/GSPD504/WT.pdf. Accessed November 1, 2015.
9. Malamed SF. Intravenous moderate sedation: rationale. In: Malamed SF, editor. Sedation: a guide to patient management. 5th edition. St Louis (MO): Mosby Elsevier; 2010. p. 274–9.
10. American Dental Association. Guidelines for the use of general anesthesia by dentists. Available at: http://www.ada.org/~/media/ADA/Member%20Center/FIles/anesthesia_guidelines.ashx. Accessed November 6, 2015.
11. Malamed SF. Intravenous sedation: complications. In: Malamed SF, editor. Sedation: a guide to patient management. 5th edition. St Louis (MO): Mosby Elsevier; 2010. p. 376–94.
12. Malamed SF. Inhalation sedation. In: Malamed SF, editor. Sedation: a guide to patient management. 5th edition. St Louis (MO): Mosby Elsevier; 2010. p. 194.
13. American Dental Association. Oral health topics: nitrous oxide. 2015. Available at: http://www.ada.org/en/member-center/oral-health-topics/nitrous-oxide. Assessed November 6, 2015.

14. Weaver JM. Why is physical restraint still acceptable for dentistry? Anesth Prog 2010;57(2):43–4. Available at: http://www.ncbi.nlm.nih.gov/pmc/articles/PMC2886916. Accessed March 31, 2016.
15. Fenton SJ. Special care in dentistry. [editorial] vol. 9; 1989. p. 183. http://onlinelibrary.wiley.com/doi/10.1111/j.1754-4505.1989.tb01183.x/abstract. Accessed November 7, 2015.
16. Oral health care for persons with disabilities: behavior management. Available at: http://paul-burtner.dental.ufl.edu/oral-health-care-for-persons-with-disabilities/providing-dental-care/specific-treatment-considerations/behavior-management/. Accessed November 7, 2015.
17. American Academy of Pediatric Dentistry. Guideline on protective stabilization for pediatric dental patients. Clinical Practice Guidelines Reference Manual 2013;37(6):194–8. Available at. http://www.aapd.org/media/policies_guidelines/g_protective.pdf. Accessed November 7, 2015.
18. Frankel RI. The papoose board® and mothers' attitudes following its use. Pediatr Dent 1991;13(5):284–8. Available at: http://www.aapd.org/assets/1/25/Frankel-13-05.pdf. Accessed October 29, 2015.
19. Murphy MG, Fields HW Jr, Machen JB. Parental acceptance of pediatric dentistry behavior management techniques. Pediatr Dent 1984;6(4):193–8. Available at: http://www.aapd.org/assets/1/25/murphy-06-04.pdf. Accessed October 29, 2015.
20. Levy H. Management of special-needs patients: there's always a way, part 2. NJAGD wisdom. Spring 2011;11(1):6–8. Available at: http://www.drhlevyassoc.com/clinicians/pubs/hlevy_theres_always_a_way_njagdwisdom_part2.pdf. Accessed November 6, 2015.
21. Yin Yang House. (CV) Conception vessel meridian – graphic. Available at: https://theory.yinyanghouse.com/acupuncturepoints/conceptionvessel_meridian_graphic. Accessed November 1, 2015.
22. A schedule of our participation courses may be found on our website. Available at: drhlevyassoc.com/clinicians.html. Accessed March 231, 2016.
23. Levy H. Dental education by circuit training. Dentaltown Magazine 2013;120:120–44. Available at: http://www.dentaltown.com/Images/Dentaltown/magimages/0713/DTJul13pg118.pdf. Accessed November 6, 2015.
24. Identafi Clinical Image Library Web site. Available at: http://www.identafi.net/tools/for-clinicians/clinical-images/15-clinical-image-library. Accessed November 1, 2015.
25. MalliDental. DentalFilm E-Speed. Video uploaded June 27, 2011. Available at: https://www.youtube.com/watch?v=60HFHwHY9Bg. Accessed November 6, 2015.
26. Tavares M, Goodson JM, Studen-Pavlovich D, et al. Reversal of soft-tissue local anesthesia with phentolamine mesylate in pediatric patients. J Am Dent Assoc 2008;139(8):1095–104.
27. Flumazenil (Rx) Romazicon. Available at: http://reference.medscape.com/drug/romazicon-flumazenil-343731. Accessed November 9, 2015.
28. United States Census Bureau. Nearly 1 in 5 people have a disability in the U.S. Census Bureau Reports. 2012. Available at: https://www.census.gov/newsroom/releases/archives/miscellaneous/cb12-134.html. Accessed November 9, 2015.
29. Levy H. Comprehensive General Dentistry in the OR, Part 1. Journal of the New York State Academy of General Dentistry, Winter 2016;6–12. Available at: https://dl.dropboxusercontent.com/u/1203452/nysagd/winter2016/index.html. Accessed April 4, 2016.

Ensuring Maintenance of Oral Hygiene in Persons with Special Needs

 CrossMark

Lisa V. Buda, DDS[a,b,c],*

KEYWORDS

- Intellectual and developmental disabilities • Maintenance • Hygiene • Caregivers
- Materials • Design • Treatment planning • General anesthesia

KEY POINTS

- Patients with intellectual and developmental disabilities who have dental needs can be treated safely and comprehensively under general anesthesia.
- There are multiple adjunctive aids that can be used to effectively complete oral hygiene for special needs patients. These include triple-headed toothbrushes, electric toothbrushes, dental waterjets, interdental brushes, foam bite blocks, and cheek retractors.
- Thoughtful treatment planning can increase the longevity of restorations and chewing table for special needs patients. Hospital-design specifications include open embrasures, flat buccal/lingual contours, and hygienic pontics with narrow chewing tables.

INTRODUCTION

Patients with special needs require modifications to treatment plans to maximize hygiene and longevity of the restoration. Although there is a broad spectrum of special needs and strategies to treat those patients, this article focuses on the special needs population that has difficulty maintaining their own oral hygiene due to intellectual and/or developmental disability (IDD) and that must be treated under general anesthesia.

Patients diagnosed with IDD present with physical and/or mental impairments before the age of 18.[1] This population is estimated at 4.6 million to 7.7 million people in the United States.[2] IDD limits the ability of patients to maintain oral hygiene or to cooperate with a dental professional, particularly when motor activity is impaired.[3] These patients may not be able to obtain dental care in a traditional setting and care must often be provided under general anesthesia. Due to a limited number of dentists practicing in this setting, the IDD population has significant issues with access to care. Examples of IDD are cerebral palsy, autism, and Down syndrome.[4]

[a] The Blende Dental Group, 390 Laurel Street, Suite 310, San Francisco, CA 94118, USA; [b] Department of Surgery, Dental Division, California Pacific Medical Center, 2333 Buchanan Street, San Francisco, CA 94115, USA; [c] Department of Surgery, Dental Division, Kaiser Permanente, 2238 Geary Boulevard, San Francisco, CA 94115, USA
* The Blende Dental Group, 390 Laurel Street, Suite 310, San Francisco, CA 94118.
E-mail address: lisabudadds@gmail.com

Dent Clin N Am 60 (2016) 593–604
http://dx.doi.org/10.1016/j.cden.2016.02.006
0011-8532/16/$ – see front matter © 2016 Elsevier Inc. All rights reserved.

CURRENT STATUS OF PATIENTS WITH INTELLECTUAL AND/OR DEVELOPMENTAL DISABILITY

The rate of untreated caries, periodontal disease, and poor oral hygiene in patients with IDD is higher than that of the general population. According to the US Centers for Disease Control and Prevention, for adults 20 years of age and older, the prevalence of untreated caries; edentulism; number of missing teeth; and mean decayed, missing, and filled teeth is higher in the population of patients with IDD than in the general population (**Table 1**).[5]

Table 1 Oral health status of population with IDD as compared to general population	General Population	Intellectual and/or Developmental Disability Population
Untreated caries	22.7%	32.2%
Edentulism	7.6%	10.9%
Mean number of missing teeth	3.6	6.7
Decayed, missing, and filled teeth mean	11.6	13.9

Data from Morgan JP, Minihan PM, Stark PC, et al. The oral health status of 4,732 adults with intellectual and developmental disabilities. J Am Dent Assoc 2012;143(8):838–46; and Beltran-Aguilar ED, Barker LK, Canto MT, et al. Surveillance for dental caries, dental sealants, tooth retention, edentulism, and enamel fluorosis: United States, 1988-1994 and 1999-2002. MMWR Surveill Summ 2005;54(3):1–43.

A 2010 systematic review of oral hygiene in those with IDD showed that although patients with intellectual disabilities had fewer filled teeth, they also have more missing and carious teeth than the general population. This may be because the chosen treatment for these patients is often extraction rather than restoration of carious teeth.[6]

It has also been shown that individuals with IDD may not have the physical ability to clean their own teeth due to lack of dexterity and understanding of the importance of proper oral hygiene.[7] Overall, a combination of poor oral hygiene, untreated caries, and treatment via extraction puts this special needs population at increased risk of pain, infection, and a decreased ability to enjoy food.

WHY TREAT IF MAINTENANCE IS AN ISSUE?

The ability to chew food is among the most basic of human needs. The National Aeronautics and Space Administration attempted to place astronauts on an all-liquid diet multiple times – all ended in failure due to the subjects' aversion to foods that they could not chew. According to food scientist Samuel Lepkovsky, soldiers given rations of potted meat "could undoubtedly survive on these rations a lot longer than we'd care to live."[8] There are multiple examples of patients who must be tube-fed yet insist on chewing food even though they must eventually spit it out. Otolaryngologist Jennifer Long has noted that patients who must make the choice between the ability to swallow food and the ability to speak often prefer to have their larynx removed specifically so that they can swallow. They prefer to be mute rather than tube-fed.[8]

Dentists serving the special needs population have the opportunity to have a significant impact on the quality of life for patients with IDD. By maximizing their occlusal table through careful treatment planning, educating caregivers, and advising a noncariogenic diet, dentists are able to preserve patients' ability to chew and enjoy food, thereby improving their quality of life.

CONSIDERATIONS FOR DENTAL TREATMENT UNDER GENERAL ANESTHESIA

Many patients with IDD can be treated safely and completely under various methods, including desensitization, therapeutic immobilization, minimal–moderate sedation, and antianxiety medications. General anesthesia is often a last resort.[9] When considering which modality to use, it is most important to evaluate the method that allows a dentist to safely treat patients to completion. This may mean recommending a treatment by another practitioner who may be able to sedate the patient if the dentist does not have the training, facilities, or experience to treat a patient. Recognizing when a referral is necessary is essential to providing the best care for special needs patients. When it comes to treating patients under general anesthesia, practitioners may elect to treat less medically complex patients in their office or surgery center with an anesthesiologist or obtain hospital privileges in their area to provide comprehensive treatment to more medically complex patients in a hospital operating room.

The evidence shows that general anesthesia is safe for special needs patients when necessary for dental rehabilitation. Studies assess risk for anesthesia based on surgical complexity and patient health status, as discussed in the American Society of Anesthesiology Physical Status classification. Dental rehabilitation is generally considered minimally invasive because it does not involve drastic changes in blood volume. Due to medical complexity in some conditions involving IDD, however, it is important to assess risk for each patient individually. Additional issues specific to patients with IDD are a limited ability to assess a patient's airway, limited ability to perform a complete history, limited ability to perform a physical examination/preoperative assessment and reliance on caregivers to ensure compliance with preanesthesia/ postanesthesia instructions due to a patient's inability to comply.[10]

Due to possible complexities and general limitations evaluating patients preoperatively, the general dentist should work closely with a team of specialists who can be available if a radiographic and full clinical examination reveals a need for treatment beyond the skills of the general dentist. This may involve having specialists on call during dental rehabilitation for suspected complex cases, ensuring that they have the appropriate training and privileges to aid with treating patients with IDD under general anesthesia in the office or in the hospital. Because it is recommended to minimize the frequency of general anesthesia, having specialists on call allows all treatment to be done in as few appointments as possible.

Overall, the most critical goal of dental treatment for special needs patients under general anesthesia is comprehensive care. This must be paired with closely monitored follow-up via a preventive program.[11] After a comprehensive appointment under general anesthesia, it is often possible for recall visits and possibly some treatment to be done under lighter sedation or modalities of restraint. Recall intervals should be determined by a patient's periodontal status and caries risk, including the ability to maintain oral hygiene in their current dental state. The literature does not address a recommended frequency of general anesthesia for dental procedures; further studies are needed. Some studies recommend general anesthesia only when there is obvious pathology. Research has shown, however, that when the recall frequency is greater than 12 months, caries rates are increased.[9]

RESTORATIVE MATERIALS

Choice of restorative material should be made with consideration for the ability of patients (or caregivers) to maintain oral hygiene, chewing habits, oral conditions with regard to chemical composition and amount of saliva and size/location of the restoration.[12] Certainly, each patient and family has different needs and abilities.

When considering dental restoration for a patient who is not cooperative with treatment awake, however, dentists must ethically choose what will provide the longest service life. Service life is determined not only by the integrity of the material but also by the design and ability of the material to prevent recurrent decay.

When it comes to choice of prosthetic material for crown or bridge restorations, a gold restoration is the most predictable choice. Marginal fit, fracture resistance, and minimal required tooth reduction result in a restoration that will provide the longest service life compared with metal-ceramic, all-ceramic, and zirconia restorations.[13] Gold was shown to have higher survival rates than metal-ceramic and all-ceramic restorations regardless of application (inlay, onlay, crown, or bridge). Secondary caries and loss of retention were the most common biological and technical reasons for failure, respectively. Material fatigue was an additional contributor to the failure of metal-ceramic and all-ceramic restorations. Full zirconia is also an attractive choice but, in comparison with gold, zirconia requires greater tooth reduction and causes more wear of the opposing tooth structure. Although gold may not be as esthetically pleasing as the available tooth-colored restorations, the advantages of material strength, compatible hardness to opposing tooth structure, and minimal tooth preparation make it an attractive choice for restoring teeth in the population of individuals with IDD who need general anesthesia for restorative care.[14]

TREATMENT PLANNING FOR PATIENTS WITH INTELLECTUAL AND/OR DEVELOPMENTAL DISABILITY

When developing a treatment plan for patients with IDD, it is important to consider the unique abilities of patients and caregivers to maintain oral hygiene and control diet. Some patients may be unable to participate in their own oral hygiene routine yet have skilled caregivers and are able to cooperate with them sufficiently to achieve good results. Others may complete their own oral hygiene poorly with no true help from caregivers. Although these 2 types of patients may present with the same dental treatment needs, their treatment plans may differ greatly to ensure a more certain prognosis. The risks, benefits, and alternatives to each treatment plan must be presented to the decision makers.

Another important aspect of developing a treatment plan for an individual with IDD involves analyzing diet. Dentists are inclined to maintain as much chewing surface as possible for patients. When a medical condition or living situation requires patients to be on a softer or pureed diet, however, dentists may choose to selectively eliminate teeth prone to infection, decay, or fracture.

There are many different theories regarding the location of the prosthetic margin and development of secondary caries. Some studies have shown that there is a lower incidence of recurrent caries on margins that are placed subgingivally due to the difference in microbial environment between the oral environment and the gingival crevice. Subgingival margin placement has been recommended for patients who have a high caries risk.[15] A systemic review and meta-analysis conducted in 2013 showed, however, that there was no significant difference in secondary caries on subgingival versus supragingival margins within 10 years. According to this study, more evidence is needed prior to recommending any particular margin placement for patients with IDD who may be at higher risk.[16] Rather, margin placement should be dictated as needed for retention and caries removal with consideration for a patient's periodontal condition.

When necessary restorative care for a person with IDD includes a bridge, dentists must ensure that it is cleansable by the patient and/or caregiver. Cast metal bridges with high-water pontics (**Fig. 1**) allow for cleansing with a toothbrush as opposed to threading floss underneath the pontic. This more predictably maintains a patient's chewing table with a bridge and requires less care than a conventional appliance.

Crown contours should be designed to facilitate cleansing with an interdental brush as opposed to necessitating the use of floss. Gingival embrasures should be kept broad and open. Restoration contours should be maximally self-cleansing as well as allowing access for oral hygiene for the caregiver.[17,18] Flat buccal and lingual contours prevent food impaction, reducing the rate of recurrent caries and periodontal disease and facilitating cleansing.[18]

To maximize the life of the restorations, occlusal tables should be kept narrow, within the confines of the root structure of the tooth, and with no obstacles in excursive movements.[19]

To simplify communication with a laboratory, laboratory slips should incorporate hospital design specifications (**Fig. 2**), for example, hygienic bridges, narrow chewing tables, and open, cleansable gingival embrasures.

ORAL HYGIENE TECHNIQUES/CAREGIVER TRAINING

Studies show that individuals with IDD have difficulty in following directions – traditional oral hygiene instructions may not be effective for this population.[4] For example, multiple studies have found that tooth brushing is most effective when done not by the patient but by a trained caregiver.[20–22] The severity of a patient's disability has been shown to correlate with higher plaque indices.[23] Consequently, one of the most important factors in improving oral health in individuals with IDD is training their caregivers adequately. Formal instruction, including lectures and hands-on training, was shown to be more effective than simply discussions on oral health.[24]

Studies show that educating caretakers in oral health and the importance of oral hygiene improves their ability to care for patients. In general, the oral health knowledge of caretakers of patients with IDD is poor. Therefore, oral health education is imperative and improves outcomes.[25] It is the responsibility of dental professionals to promote

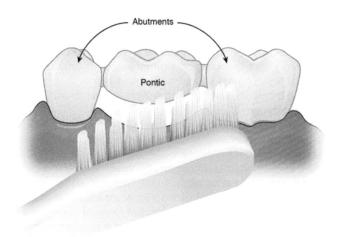

Fig. 1. Hygienic bridge.

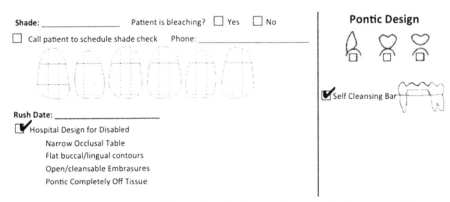

Fig. 2. Laboratory slip. (*Adapted from* The Blende Dental Group, San Francisco, CA.)

oral health education in the community of caregivers to allow patients better outcomes.

The choice of oral hygiene instruments can offer a significant improvement to hygiene. Electric toothbrushes have been shown to remove more plaque than single-headed or triple-headed toothbrushes.[22] There are a wide variety of these brushes available. Two of the most popular brands of brushes are the Philips Sonicare and Oral-B Electric toothbrushes. The former has an oval vibrating head of various sizes whereas the latter has a round oscillating head. Some patients may object to the sound and feel of electric toothbrushes, but, due to their effectiveness, they should be considered for use by caregivers of patients with IDD.

If electric toothbrushes cannot be used, a manual triple-headed toothbrush, which is designed to simultaneously clean the buccal, lingual, and occlusal tooth surfaces, has been shown more effective than a traditional single-headed toothbrush in reducing plaque scores and gingivitis.[20,23,26] Examples of such brushes are the Surround Toothbrush from Specialized Care (**Fig. 3**) and the Dr. Barman's Superbrush. Nurses preferred brushing cerebral palsy patients' teeth with a triple-headed toothbrush over a single-headed toothbrush. They also required fewer additional instructions over time when brushing with a triple-headed brush. The advantages were seen as a reduction in the time needed for brushing, reduced stimulation of the gag reflex, and decreased bleeding. Most issues from brushing with the single-headed brush were related to not spending enough time in any particular area of the mouth and difficulty with brushing the lingual surfaces of the teeth. Lingual plaque scores were reduced by a factor of 2 when using the triple-headed brush versus the traditional single-headed toothbrush.[23]

Use of a triple-headed brush may not be effective in patients with periodontal disease. This is because the brush may not be able to appropriately cleanse the buccal and lingual surfaces for these patients.[27]

Although various toothbrush designs can effectively remove plaque from the buccal, lingual, and occlusal surfaces of teeth, tooth brushing alone cannot penetrate the interproximal surfaces. Interdental brushes (**Fig. 4**) are a suitable alternative to flossing for patients with IDD due to the brushes' effective removal of plaque and relative ease of use. Various diameters of interdental brushes are available to accommodate differences in embrasure size.[28,29] Depending on patient cooperation, floss handles can also be a useful adjunct. They should be used in a manner similar to conventional floss, with the handle eliminating the need for 2-handed manipulation.

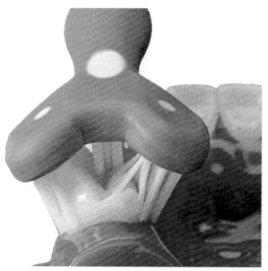

Fig. 3. Triple-headed brush. (*Courtesy of* Specialized Care Co, Inc, Hampton, NH, with permission.)

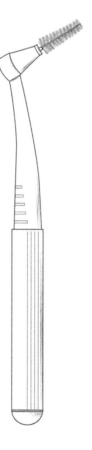

Fig. 4. Interdental brush.

Yet another flossing alternative is the dental waterjet (**Fig. 5**). Studies have shown that a dental waterjet, when combined with a manual or electric toothbrush, is as effective as a manual toothbrush and floss at removing plaque and reducing gingivitis.[30] There are multiple studies that have found the dental waterjet a suitable alternative to flossing.[31]

Patients with IDD do not always cooperate during the oral hygiene routine. Two commonalities are a reluctance to maintain their mouth in the open position and strong lip tone preventing visual inspection of the teeth. There are several adjunct tools caregivers can use to coax patients into cooperating. For example, insertion and careful rotation of a foam bite block or the use of a Molt mouth prop can help disclude the teeth (**Figs. 6** and **7**).

Anecdotal evidence shows that patients with developmental disabilities tend to have strong lower lips.[4] Wet metal retractors (often conventionally used for dental photography **Fig. 8**) may be used to retract the patients' cheeks and allow for visual inspection or oral hygiene access. Care must be taken to do this gently and it may only be suitable for a subset of patients, because the metal retractor may cause injury with sudden movement.

DIET

Dental caries is caused by a process involving factors within a host (tooth surface, saliva flow and composition, and bacteria) and the host's diet. Frequency of intake of cariogenic foods and drinks, notably carbohydrates, is the major factor in causing

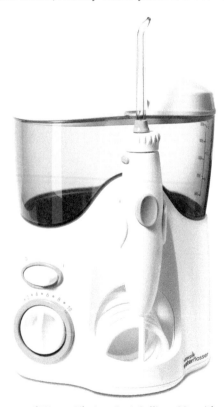

Fig. 5. Waterjet. (*Courtesy of* Water Pik, Inc, Fort Collins, CO, with permission.)

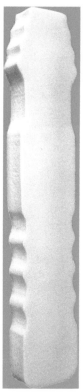

Fig. 6. Foam bite block. (*Courtesy of* Specialized Care Co, Inc, Hampton, NH, with permission.)

tooth decay. Oral bacteria produce acids by metabolizing these carbohydrates, thus allowing minerals to diffuse out of the tooth, leading to caries.[32]

Patients living in group settings often have the benefit of receiving structured meals with controlled consumption of refined carbohydrates.[33–35] For all patients with IDD, a noncariogenic diet should be discussed with caregivers. If it is medically necessary for a patient to consume a diet rich in carbohydrates (for weight gain), the dental professional should counsel caregivers on the importance of reducing frequency and duration of carbohydrate consumption and preventive strategies.[36]

SUMMARY

Maintenance of oral hygiene in persons with special needs has been discussed in the context of treatment planning to explicitly ensure that maintenance and oral hygiene could be more easily maintained while providing patients with a sufficient chewing table. Methods for gaining access to these patients mouths via retractors and bite blocks with the use of triple-headed or electric toothbrushes for maximum plaque removal is a crucial element to ensuring that the dentition of persons with IDD can be maintained. Finally, surveying their diet for frequency of carbohydrate consumption allows making the mechanical hygiene work simpler by reducing the amount of cariogenic substances these patients consume.

With these tools, special needs patients can have better oral health outcomes and can be kept chewing longer. And, as eloquently stated by Vietnamese Zen Monk Thich

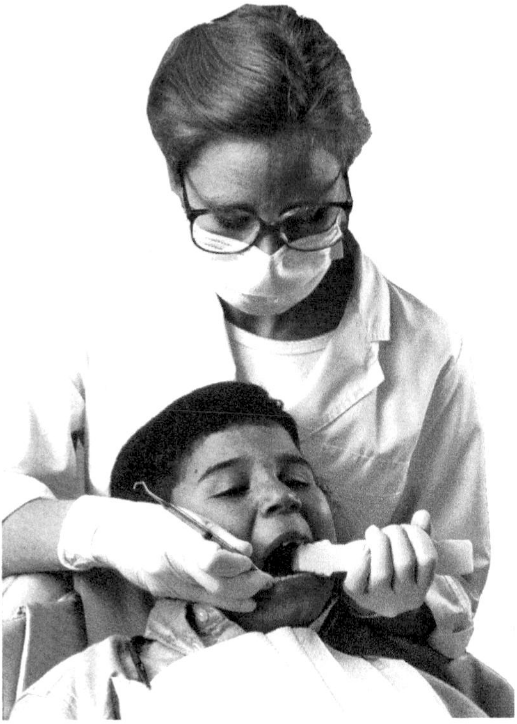

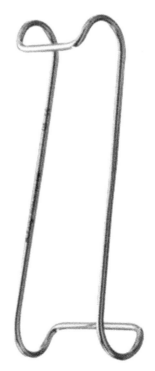

Fig. 7. Use of foam bite block. (*Courtesy of* Specialized Care Co, Inc, Hampton, NH, with permission.)

Fig. 8. Metal cheek retractor.

Nhat Hanh, by helping them chew, dentists have the power to make these patients innately happier.

If you truly get in touch with a piece of carrot, you get in touch with the soil, the rain, the sunshine. You get in touch with Mother Earth and eating in such a way, you feel in touch with true life, your roots, and that is meditation. If we "chew" every morsel of our food in that way we become grateful and when you are grateful, you are happy [author's emphasis].

REFERENCES

1. FAQ on intellectual disability. American Association on Intellectual and Developmental Disabilities Web site. Available at: http://aaidd.org/intellectual-disability/definition/faqs-on-intellectual-disability#.VdEr_RNViko. Accessed August 16, 2015.
2. How Prevalent are Intellectual and Developmental Disabilities in the United States? Bethesda Institute Web site. Available at: http://flroof.org/publication/view/how-prevalent-are-intellectual-and-developmental-disabilities-in-the-united-states/. Accessed August 16, 2015.
3. Oredugba FA, Akindayomi Y. Oral health status and treatment needs of children and young adults attending a day centre for individuals with special health care needs. BMC Oral Health 2008;8:30.
4. Shin CJ, Saeed S. Toothbrushing barriers for people with developmental disabilities: a pilot study. Spec Care Dentist 2013;33(6):269–74.
5. Morgan JP, Minihan PM, Stark PC, et al. The oral health status of 4,732 adults with intellectual and developmental disabilities. J Am Dent Assoc 2012;143(8):838–46.
6. Anders PL, Davis EL. Oral health of patients with intellectual disabilities: a systematic review. Spec Care Dentist 2010;30(3):110–7.
7. Geganegi KS, Tandon S. Tooth surface protection for individuals who are mentally disabled. Spec Care Dentist 2008;28(1):32–8.
8. Roach M. Gulp: adventures on the alimentary canal. 1st edition. New York: W. W. Norton & Company; 2013.
9. Dougherty N. The dental patient with special needs: a review of indications for treatment under general anesthesia. Spec Care Dentist 2009;29(1):17–20.
10. Messieha Z, Ananda RC, Hoffman I, et al. Five year outcomes study of dental rehabilitation conducted under general anesthesia for special needs patients. Anesth Prog 2007;54(4):170–4.
11. Mallineni SK, Yiu CKY. A retrospective review of outcomes of dental treatment performed for special needs patients under general anaesthesia: 2 year follow-up. ScientificWorldJournal 2014;2014:748353, 6 pages.
12. ADA Council on Scientific Affairs. Direct and indirect restorative materials. J Am Dent Assoc 2003;134:463–72.
13. Wirz J, Jager K. 1st edition. Evaluation of commonly used crown systems. Quintessence of dental technology, vol. 22. Hanover Park (IL): Quintessence Publ. Comp. Inc; 1999.
14. Schwass DR, Lyons KM, Purton DG. How long with it last? The expected longevity of prosthodontics and restorative treatment. N Z Dent J 2013;109(3):98–105.
15. Molin M, Bergman B, Ericson A. A clinical evaluation of conical crown retained dentures. J Prosthet Dent 1993;70(3):251–6.
16. Papageorgiou SN, Papadelli AP, Koidis PT, et al. The effect of prosthetic margin location on caries susceptibility. A systemic review and meta-analysis. Br Dent J 2013;214(12):617–24.

17. Singh Y, Saini M. Designing crown contour in fixed prosthodontics: a neglected area. Ann essences dent 2011;3(1):142–7.
18. Becker CM, Kaldahl WB. Crown contours that promote access for oral hygiene. Quintessence Int Dent Dig 1981;12(2):233–8.
19. Schneider DM. Full coverage temporization – an outline of goals, methods and uses (III). Quintessence Int Dent Dig 1980;11(5):31–8.
20. Weddell JA, Sanders BJ, Jones JE. Dental problems of children with disabilities. In: McDonald RE, Avery DR, Dean JA, editors. Dentistry for the child and adolescent. 8th edition. Philadelphia: Mosby; 2004. p. 526–30, 543–6.
21. Rodrigues dos Santos MT, Masiero D, Novo NF, et al. Oral conditions in children with cerebral palsy. J Dent Child (Chic) 2003;70(1):40–6.
22. Doğan MC, Alaçam A, Aşici N, et al. Clinical evaluation of the plaque-removing ability of three different toothbrushes in a mentally disabled group. Acta Odontol Scand 2004;62(6):350–4.
23. Yitzhak M, Sarnat H, Rakocz M, et al. The effect of toothbrush design on the ability of nurses to brush the teeth of institutionalized cerebral palsy patients. Spec Care Dentist 2013;33(1):20–7.
24. Gonzalez EE, Nathe CN, Logothetis DD, et al. Training caregivers: disabilities and dental hygiene. Int J Dent Hyg 2013;11(4):293–7.
25. Khanagar S, Kumar A, Rajanna V, et al. Oral health care education and its effect on caregivers' knowledge, attitudes, and practices: a randomized controlled trial. J Int Soc Prev Community Dent 2014;4(2):122–8.
26. Zimmer S, Didner B, Roulet JF. Clinical study on the plaque removing ability of new triple headed toothbrush. J Clin Periodontol 1999;26:281–5.
27. Levin L, Marom Y, Ashkenazi M. Brushing skills and plaque reduction using single- and triple-headed toothbrushes. Quintessence Int 2012;43(6):525–31.
28. Imai PH, Yu X, MacDonald D. Comparison of interdental brush to dental floss for reduction of clinical parameters of periodontal disease: a systematic review. Can J Dent Hyg 2012;46(1):63–79.
29. Seidel-Bittke D. Caring for the developmentally disabled: tips on providing needed care to special patients. Waco,Texas: RDH; 2005. p. 32–6.
30. Barnes CM, Russell CM, Reinhardt RA, et al. Comparison of irrigation to floss as an adjunct to tooth brushing: effect on bleeding, gingivitis and supragingival plaque. J Clin Dent 2005;1(3):71–7.
31. Jahn CA. The dental water jet: a historical review of the literature. J Dent Hyg 2010;84(3):114–20.
32. Galhotra V, Sofat A, Dua H, et al. Anticariogenic and cariostatic potential of components of diet: a review. Indian J Dental Sci 2014;6(4):79–85.
33. Gabre P, Martinsson T, Gahnberg L. Incidence of, and reasons for, tooth mortality among mentally retarded adults during a 10-year period. Acta Odontol Scand 1999;57(1):55–61.
34. Rodríguez Vázquez C, Garcillan R, Rioboo R, et al. Prevalence of dental caries in an adult population with mental disabilities in Spain. Spec Care Dentist 2002; 22(2):65–9.
35. Steinberg AD, Zimmerman S. The Lincoln dental caries study: a three-year evaluation of dental caries in persons with various mental disorders. J Am Dent Assoc 1978;97(6):981–4.
36. American Academy of Pediatric Dentistry. Council on Clinical Affairs. Guideline on management of dental patients with special health care needs. Pediatr Dent 2012;34(5):160–5.

Evidence-based Dentistry and Its Role in Caring for Special Needs Patients

 CrossMark

Alan N. Queen, DDS, FAGD*

KEYWORDS

- Evidence-based dentistry • Special care dentistry • Special needs dentistry
- Treatment accommodations

KEY POINTS

- Special needs dentistry is frequently misconstrued to refer only to patients with mental or developmental disabilities. Those with physical, medical, and/or psychological disabilities also have special needs that may require accommodations in dental care.
- Studies by the US Census Bureau indicate that about 1 in 8 people in the United States have some form of disability that would affect the way they care for their teeth and/or would pose a barrier to their receiving dental care.
- Evidence-based dentistry (EBD) is a concept ideally suited and applicable to special needs dentistry. As the special needs of patients varies according to the individual, so should the way we evaluate our patient, prescribe a course of treatment, and implement that treatment plan.
- Many medical conditions can also present barriers to care or complications to consider in preparing a treatment plan. Using EBD, these issues need to be addressed to develop a personalized treatment plan.

"No good! Do it over!" the instructor bellowed at the dental student in a preclinical laboratory 30 years ago. The student's offense was deviating, ever so slightly, from "core technique," the rigid, one-size-fits-all way of doing dentistry.

Like G.V. Black's "extension for prevention"[1] method of operative dentistry, this rigid concept of performing dental procedures was taught for more than a century to generations of dentists. Today, dentists are embracing "evidence-based dentistry" (EBD) as a means of coping with variations in the dental patient population, something that is especially prevalent among special needs patients.

Special needs dentistry is frequently misconstrued to refer only to patients with mental or developmental disabilities. Although these patients certainly do have special needs, the category includes far more than these patients alone.[2]

Conflict of Interest Disclosure: The author has nothing to disclose.
Department of Dental and Oral Medicine, New York Presbyterian/Queens Medical Center, 56-45 Main Street, Flushing, NY 11355, USA
* 45-10 Kissena Boulevard (#PR2), Flushing, NY 11355.
E-mail address: Queensdentist@aol.com

Studies by the US Census Bureau[3] show that approximately 1 in 8 people in the United States have some form of disability that would affect the way they care for their teeth or would pose a barrier to their receiving dental care.[4] These disabilities can be physical, such as manual dexterity or mobility issues afflicting patients with stroke or Parkinson disease, victims of severe car accidents, or battlefield wounds in returning soldiers.

Other patients with special needs may have medical factors affecting their care. Patients undergoing radiation and/or chemotherapy for cancer, patients with diabetes (especially those whose disease is poorly controlled), patients with human immuno-deficiency virus, and the frail elderly may have multiple medical issues that present barriers to care and contraindications to "business as usual" dentistry.

There are also mental and psychological considerations for some special needs patients that need to be addressed. Patients with mental retardation, autism, or various psychiatric disorders may be unable to care for themselves or even give their own consent for treatment, and require deviation from "core technique" as well.

EVIDENCE-BASED DENTISTRY

According to the American Dental Association, "EBD is a patient-centered approach to treatment decisions, which provides personalized dental care based on the most current scientific knowledge."[5] This is a radical departure from the traditional way of teaching dentistry that most dental schools used for more than a century.

Generations of dentists have taken licensing board examinations on live patients where they were frequently penalized for deviating even slightly from the ideal preparation espoused by G.V. Black more than a century ago. Black published his concepts in his *Manual of Operative Dentistry* in 1896, including his concept of "extension for prevention." This called for extending cavity preparations into healthy tooth structure to eliminate grooves, pits, and fissures that allegedly could decay later. His theory was to remove these otherwise healthy tooth structures now before they could decay in the future. This was how dentistry was taught well into the 1980s.

However, more recent studies have shown that needlessly extending cavity preparations actually weakens teeth, and this concept is no longer taught in dental schools today. This is an example of how EBD has changed clinical practice.

EBD has also changed the way practitioners evaluate their patients from the minute they walk in the operatory door. No longer are the patients just "teeth attached to a body," where the focus is solely on the mouth. Research has shown that there are a myriad of medical conditions that affect the teeth and oral health, sometimes increasing the risk of caries, predisposing a patient to development of periodontal disease, or changing the prognosis for success of dental procedures, such as implants. There are also dental conditions that can have systemic effects on the body, including periodontal disease and untreated dental infections. Inability to masticate properly can affect nutrition, with far-ranging sequelae.

MEDICAL EVALUATION OF THE DENTAL PATIENT

Not so very long ago, in the 1970s, the medical evaluation of dental patients was usually a cursory medical history that was intended primarily to screen for the need to premedicate a patient with prophylactic antibiotics and avoid medication interactions with local anesthesia.

However, over the intervening years, the link between systemic health and oral health has become a subject of much research. Linkages between periodontal disease and cardiovascular issues (including heart attack and stroke) have been the subject of many studies. The role of inflammation in periodontal disease and its systemic health affects also has been a hot topic.

Patients with special needs often present with multiple medical problems, so the effects and side-effects of the medications taken must be evaluated not just on the initial visit, but routinely at each visit to account for changes that may have been made between dental visits.

Bisphosphonates and their role in osteonecrosis of the jaw is also a hot topic in dental research, as practitioners have recognized the effects of medications taken by patients on their oral health. Lists of drugs that cause xerostomia have lengthened over the years, and xerostomia treatments are now even advertised on television to the public.

Anticoagulant treatments are much more common, as the use of coated cardiac stents has increased over the past 20 years, and patients undergo life-saving surgeries for medical problems that would have been fatal in prior years. Some patients present taking 1 or more anticoagulating agents, ranging from simple aspirin to warfarin (Coumadin), clopidogrel (Plavix), and others. Any dental treatment that could involve bleeding, including a simple dental prophylaxis, must be treatment planned with these issues in mind.

Many medical conditions can also present barriers to care or complications to consider in preparing a treatment plan. Using EBD, these issues need to be addressed to develop a personalized treatment plan.

Also, because patients with special needs may not be able to advocate for themselves, and caregivers may not be fully informed of a patient's detailed medical history, it is important to coordinate dental treatment with their physicians. Medical clearance for dental treatment should be obtained from the physician, especially before invasive procedures, such as oral surgery, are performed.

PHYSICAL EVALUATION OF THE DENTAL PATIENT

Basic considerations, such as can patients brush their teeth on their own? Do they have limited manual dexterity? Or are they paraplegic and thus rely on others for their oral hygiene? Should a patient with oral hygiene issues be treatment planned for a complex fixed prosthetic restoration that will be difficult to maintain, or would something removable be a wiser choice? Even the choice of design for a removable prosthesis can be fraught with issues for those with limited manual dexterity who have insufficient help at home. What is "ideal" for one patient may not be ideal for another.

Another physical factor to consider is whether patients sit in the dental chair. And if so, can they be reclined, or must they be treated in an upright position? Do they use an oxygen tank to help them breathe, and will that pose a problem? For example, using an open flame in an operatory (ie, to soften wax, border mold a tray, or sear off the end of a gutta percha point) is not wise if the patient is on oxygen.

The issue of duration of treatment also should be considered. Long procedures, requiring a patient to keep his or her mouth open for extended periods of time, can be very difficult for a developmentally disabled or frail elderly patient. It might be necessary to pick a different treatment if the patient does not have the stamina or ability to cooperate for longer stretches of time.

Dividing treatment into more, shorter appointments can sometime be the answer. Preparing fixed bridge abutments 1 per session rather than all at once could be considered. Preparing a tooth, placing a temporary filling, and then completing the restoration at the next appointment could be another needed accommodation that could be treatment planned.

EVIDENCE-BASED DENTISTRY: ADJUSTING TREATMENT ACCOMMODATIONS TO FIT THE PATIENT'S NEEDS

Because the range of needs varies widely, the range of care available must address the problems as well. The levels of care offered can be broadly divided into 3 levels:

1. Those patients with minimal barriers to care who can be treated in a normal clinic setting with minimal accommodations needed.
2. Those patients who can be treated in a normal clinic setting but who require a higher level of accommodations to manage their physical, behavioral, and/or psychological disabilities.
3. Those patients who cannot be treated in a normal clinical setting because of behavioral, psychological, medical, and/or physical disabilities. These patients need to be treated in a hospital operating room (OR), under intravenous or general anesthesia with appropriate monitoring.

Each patient should be assessed at the initial visit to determine his or her needed level of care. This should be constantly reassessed as treatment progresses. A thorough medical history, including a list of all medications, should be taken at the initial visit and medical clearance obtained from the patient's physician. This should be updated periodically as well as before any invasive procedures.

Level 1: Minimal Accommodations Needed for Treatment

Most Level 1 patients can be treated anywhere, including a private dental office. These could be patients who have mild developmental disabilities, such as high-functioning patients with Down syndrome, very elderly patients with debilitating medical or psychiatric conditions such as chronic obstructive pulmonary disease or advanced emphysema, post-stroke patients, or patients with mild to moderate dementia. Many elderly patients present with a number of concurrent chronic conditions that must be addressed as well. General practice residents should graduate with the skills and confidence needed to treat these patients in their private offices.[6]

Treatment accommodations can range from seating the patient in a more upright position during treatment to aide breathing, breaks in treatment to reduce stress, using "tell-show-do" to continually reorient a patient who may be confused or anxious, shorter appointments (usually in the morning when the patient is more well-rested), and modifying treatment plans to address physical and mental limitations.[7] Treatment can be provided in a wheelchair for those who cannot be readily transferred to the dental chair (**Fig. 1**).

Level 2: Moderate Accommodations Needed for Treatment

Level 2 patients are those whose behavior and/or physical limitations require more substantial management. For example, a nonverbal developmentally disabled patient may require premedication with an oral sedative for treatment to be possible. A papoose (**Fig. 2**) may be needed in some cases. Other patients may require additional staff to be present during treatment to hold a head up, retract tongue and/or lips, or to hold the patient's hand for both comfort and to prevent sudden grabbing of the dentist and/or assistant during treatment.

The least restrictive environment is usually the best for the patient. Many developmentally disabled patients can be treated without physical restraints, sometimes using mild oral presedation. For safety purposes, it is usually advisable to defer to the patient's physician to write the sedative prescription so there is less likelihood of a drug interaction or other issue, especially because many of these medically

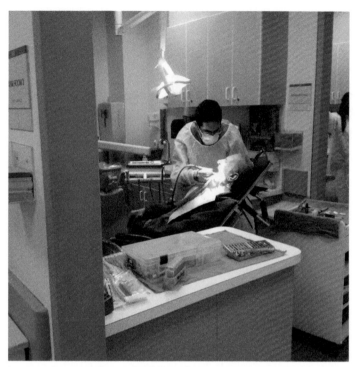

Fig. 1. Patients can be treated in a wheelchair, if necessary, when they are unable to transfer to a dental chair.

compromised patients are on multiple medications concurrently that could be changed at any time. Often, the presence of a caregiver in the operatory during treatment aides in calming an anxious patient. If a papoose is required, it should be used for the minimum amount of time necessary to complete treatment.

Level 3: High Level of Accommodations Needed for Treatment

Level 3 patients are those for whom treatment in a normal clinical setting is impossible. This may be due to medical or physical impairment, or because of psychological or mental considerations. A patient with Parkinson disease with uncontrolled tremors requiring extensive operative dentistry may not be able to be safely treated in a dental office or clinic. A severely debilitated elderly patient requiring oral surgery may need to be hospitalized, even if only for a few hours on the day of the procedure. Severely developmentally disabled patients, some of whom may refuse to even enter a dental operatory, making using a papoose impossible, may need to be treated in the OR as well.

Experienced clinicians regularly take patients with special needs to the OR for treatment when required, and are sometimes assisted by dental residents in rendering that treatment. However, because of the risks inherent in general anesthesia, as well as the higher costs and restrictions by Medicaid and other insurers, this type of treatment modality is usually kept as a last resort and is not used merely to perform a routine 6-month recall examination and/or cleaning, for example.

Some hospitals have both the equipment and staff to perform comprehensive dental treatment in the OR while the patient is under general anesthesia. For some

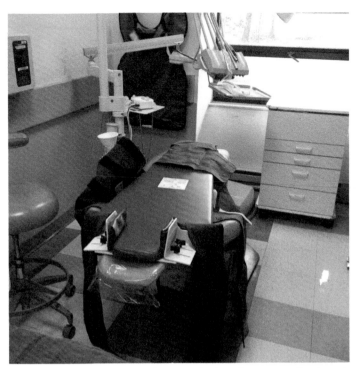

Fig. 2. Use of a papoose may be required to provide dental treatment for the safety of both the patient and the personnel providing treatment. The least restrictive method of treatment is usually the best.

of these patients, it may have been years, if ever, since they have had their dental needs treated. Radiographs, examinations, and the full range of dental procedures, from operative dentistry and oral surgery to periodontal treatment, can be performed in the OR.[2]

OTHER TREATMENT CONSIDERATIONS

By the nature of their impairment, most of these patients are not candidates for orthodontic or complex prosthodontic treatment, especially those on Level 3. But the OR gives the treating dentist the ability to both address acute issues, and to stabilize the remaining dentition where possible, to permit the patient to function. Comprehensive care is rendered during the OR session so that the patient will not need a return trip for treatment for as long as possible.

The treatment plan must address the accommodation level, as well as the nature and extent of the disability or disabilities present. Obviously, a Level 2 patient who cannot tolerate an alginate impression will not be a candidate for a removable partial denture. Dentists must be able to make real-world judgments and alter their "ideal" treatment plans accordingly.

Last, it is necessary to address the patient's home care regimen, especially in cases in which caries and/or periodontal disease is detected. Many times, an electric toothbrush can do wonders to improve oral hygiene. Supplemental fluoride, in the form of rinses or toothpaste, can help, subject to the patient's ability to comply with rinsing and then expectorating rather than swallowing the fluoride agent.

SUMMARY

EBD is a concept ideally suited and applicable to the field of special needs dentistry. As the special needs of patients varies according to the individual, so should the way we evaluate our patient, prescribe a course of treatment, and implement that treatment plan.

Future generations of dental students and residents should be trained in these concepts not just for treatment of patients with special needs, but for the general patient population as well. It is imperative that the dental community not retreat in the face of what many deem to be "difficult" patients with special needs. Knowledge and training can overcome many barriers to treatment. Where necessary, hospital-based facilities should be available nationwide for treatment of patients not able to be treated in a normal clinic setting. Training should be made available, both as postgraduate continuing education courses and through dental residency programs, to enable all dentists to provide the treatment our patients require.

REFERENCES

1. Joseph R. The father of modern dentistry–Dr. Greene Vardiman Black (1836-1915). J Conserv Dent 2005;8:5–6.
2. Queen AN. Trouble for special needs dentistry. Newsday. September 14, 2015;76(No. 12):A25.
3. Brault MW. "Americans with disabilities: 2005" current population reports. United States Government: US Census Bureau; 2008.
4. Waldman HB. Preparing dental graduates to provide care to individuals with special needs. J Dent Educ 2005;69(2):249–54.
5. American Dental Association. Available at: https://ebd.ada.org/en/about/. Accessed April 13, 2015.
6. American Dental Association Commission on Dental Accreditation. 2004.
7. Saint Louis, Catherine. Dentists open a closed door for autism. New York Times October 20, 2014; p. 1.

The Dental Needs and Treatment of Patients with Down Syndrome

 CrossMark

Azizah Bin Mubayrik, BDS, MSc, Clin Cert.

KEYWORDS

- Down syndrome • Oral health • Dental management • Systemic considerations

KEY POINTS

- Down syndrome is associated with various systemic findings, oral findings, and diseases.
- Oral health can be maintained through proper knowledge, regular visits, and proper intervention.
- Dentists need to take a holistic approach including behavioral, oral, and systemic issues.
- This review of the literature focuses on oral anomalies, systemic interaction, management, and recommendations.

INTRODUCTION

Down syndrome (DS) is the most common chromosomal disorder and cause of mental retardation. First described by Esquirol in 1838, and later in 1866, this disorder was described by John Langdon Down and named mongolism.[1–3] It is caused by an extra copy of chromosome 21, giving a chromosome count of 47.[1] Trisomy 21 results from nondisjunction of homologous chromosomes 21 during gametogenesis or early after fertilization.[4,5] It occurs most frequently (90%) during meiosis in women. The remaining percentage arises from the father's side or from nondisjunction of chromosomes during a postzygotic mitosis. Maternal age plays a role in the nondisjunction of chromosome 21.[6,7]

Robertsonian translocation to another acrocentric chromosome or isochromosome, usually chromosome 14t(14q;21q) or t(21q;21q). The affected child has 3 copies of the long arm of chromosome 21 instead of 2. In 25% of the cases, one of the parents is trait carrier.[6,7]

Mosaicism is a form of DS in which an individual has 2 or more genetically distinct cell lines, some with the normal number of chromosomes, and some that are aneuploid. It is caused by a nondisjunction during postzygotic mitosis.[6,7]

Conflicts of Interest: The author declares that there is conflicts of interest.
Department Oral Medicine & Diagnostic Sciences, College of Dentistry, King Saud University, Riyadh, Saudi Arabia
E-mail address: aalmobeirik@ksu.edu.sa

Regardless of the chromosomal abnormality background, individuals with DS have a noninherited mental retardation with varying range of cognitive dysfunction and characteristic facial features. General features include cardiovascular defects, skeletal abnormalities, ocular defects, protuberant abdomen, hypogonadism, and delayed puberty. Craniofacial features may include brachycephaly, flat occiput, broad and short neck, hypoplasia of the maxilla, upslanting palpebral fissures, short ears, and small chin. Some of the oral manifestations are periodontal disease, delayed eruption, malocclusion, thickening of lips, macroglossia, and fissured and protruding tongue.

DENTAL CARIES IN INDIVIDUALS WITH DOWN SYNDROME

It is generally agreed that caries prevalence and incidence in both institutionalized and noninstitutionalized individuals with DS is lower than in normal and other mentally retarded individuals.[8–12] A meta-analysis revealed that individuals with DS have significantly lower levels of dental caries.[13] Causes for low caries levels are delayed eruption, spacing of teeth, congenital oligodontia, and some salivary characteristics.[14–16] Small teeth and morphologic anomalies may also play a role.[16–18] A few reports showed higher or no difference in caries level in individuals with DS.[9,13,19,20] Differences in results could be attributed to sample characteristics such as sociodemographic and geographic location. Other risk factors are sweets intake, fluoridation, poor oral hygiene, frequency of dental checkups, deficiency of health education, lack of prevention programs, and the awareness of the parents.[10,15,20–24] Extent of disability and intelligence quotient (IQ) level also influenced oral health status.[21]

PERIODONTAL DISEASES

Patients with DS have increased prevalence of early progressive periodontitis and edentulism compared with normal or mentally retarded individuals.[15,24–26] Severe periodontitis usually occurs during teenage years, with more bone loss than other mentally retarded patients.[27] The average rate of bone resorption is 0.03 mm/y, with severe bone loss in 65% by 35 years of age, primarily affecting the lower anterior area.[27] Both local and systemic factors have been suggested to cause periodontal destruction. Local causes may include reduced oral hygiene, calculus deposits, macroglossia, tooth morphology, gingival tissue abnormalities, saliva characteristics.[28,29] Another factor is the differences in subgingival microbiota among patients with DS.[29,30] For example, there is an increased level of *Propionibacterium acnes* (associated with persistent apical periodontal infections), *Treponema socranskii* (linked to tissue destruction), and *Streptococcus constellatus* (refractory periodontitis).[30]

Systemic factors are DS related, such as oxidative burst intensity of granulocytes and monocytes, depressed chemotaxis, impaired oxidative metabolism, and immunity.[28,29,31–35] Another possible cause is decreased CD4+/CD8+ ratio, and thus altered immune regulation and function.[36]

Poor periodontal health and prognosis have been linked to individual age, IQ level, and parental education.[37] However, supervised brushing, good dental care, and prevention measures tend to improve the periodontal status.[32,37–41]

Properties of Saliva

Studies, although not conclusive, have reported variations in flow rate, pH and salivary electrolyte levels (sodium, potassium, chloride, calcium, phosphorous), α-amylases, buffering capacity, and salivary counts of mutans streptococci.[14–16,42–44] The lower predominance of caries in patients with DS is correlated with higher levels of immuno-globulin A in saliva.[45]

Total antioxidant capacity is a salivary factor known to be inversely related to caries, and it is significantly lower in DS, whereas sialic acid level is higher than that of normal controls.[46–50] An increased level of superoxide dismutase was observed in the saliva of patients with DS inducing the accumulation of hydrogen peroxide, which can cause oxidative damage.[51]

Patients with DS had increased pH and sodium bicarbonate levels in their pa-rotid saliva, which may be one of the factors responsible for the reduced incidence of dental caries noted in these persons. Salivary enzymes also were altered in persons with DS.[16,52]

OCCLUSAL AND DENTAL ANOMALIES

The most frequent occlusal abnormalities are caused by variations in vertical and hor-izontal dimensions such as open bite, crossbite, and extreme overjet, with a higher prevalence of class III (pseudoprogeny).[53–56] Congenitally missing teeth and delayed tooth eruption are seen more among patients with DS.[57,58] The most common tooth agenesis is of the third molars, followed by maxillary lateral incisors and second pre-molars.[59–61] In some cases supernumerary teeth are encountered.[61]

Morphologic diversity such as microdontia and peg laterals are common findings among patients with DS.[62] In general, all the teeth, with the exception of lower incisors and upper first molars, are smaller than normal.[60] In many cases of DS, the maxillary canine and premolars are impacted.[59] Another reported morphologic abnormality is taurodontism, and this has been attributed to slow mitosis in DS.[63,64]

CRANIOFACIAL COMPLEX

In general, the craniofacial complex is smaller than in normal individuals, with brachy-cephaly, cranial base flattening, small sella turcica, and prominent forehead. The cranial bones are thin and diploë is absent.[55,65] Paranasal sinuses and supraorbital ridges are missing or underdeveloped.[55,65] Similarly, nasal bone agenesis or incom-plete calcification is occasionally seen among the younger age groups.[55,65] The nasal bone is shorter and angled acutely, with an underdeveloped frontal process of the maxilla, which gives the appearance of middle face retrusion.[55,65] The growth of both jaws is reduced.[62] The mandibular ramus and body are short. The vertical dimen-sions of the maxillary and mandibular alveolar height are reduced.[66]

SOFT TISSUE AND OROFACIAL ANOMALIES

Soft tissue characteristics include fissured, protrusive, and scalloped tongue. The fissures are mainly on the dorsal surface of the anterior two-thirds of the tongue with different shapes and pattern.[67,68] There is macroglossia, and dry tongue dorsum is caused by mouth breathing. Everted lower lip,[68] lack of lip seal, drool-ing, and angular cheilitis are common features among these patients. They are also prone to congenital structural anomalies such as bifid uvula, and submucous cleft lip and palate.[67–69]

The protruding tongue and muscle hypotonia can lead to oral motor problems such as speech impairment, mouth breathing, inaccurate and slow tongue movement, and difficulty in mastication and swallowing.[60,69]

The severity and development of hypotonicity may vary among persons with DS. Muscle, ligament, and joints laxity lead to nonphysiologic gait, drooling, and can compromise the periodontal ligaments.[55,70] People with DS are also prone to have agenesis one of the salivary glands.[71,72]

DENTAL CARE
Dental Care Access

In spite of the way that individuals with DS have a greater need of dental care, they have difficulty getting expert consideration. Absence of parental awareness that their children have dental issues, children's fears, and parents' difficulty in finding oral health care are among the reasons for this.

Lack of knowledge and training of caregivers may also play a role.[24,73,74]

Communication

Language delay and impairment in DS is a major barrier to effective communication, and social interaction and development. Children with DS thus tend to depend on nonverbal skills for longer periods than typical children. These patients are likely to have language deficits, particularly in expressive language, and poor speech intelligibility.[75,76]

Anxiety has its own effects on the communication process. It is advisable to interview patients away from the stimuli of the dental setting and to allow time for reflection, questions, and interaction.[77] Starting the meeting by building up a good rapport can reduce the anxiety, distractions, and so forth.

It is a good practice to direct the interview to the patient. This practice assesses the patient's ability to communicate, establish rapport, and gains the patient's confidence. Abstain from correcting them or finishing sentences for them. Exercise gentle persistence and do not try to represent them. If you do not understand what a patient is trying to say, ask the patient to rephrase it and ask for confirmation that it is right. Whenever possible, short inquiries that require short answers, or a gesture or a shake of the head, are to be used. Interviewers must consider that inability is regularly associated with shame. Like all individuals, individuals with inabilities prefer not to be seen as unfit, inept, or inferior. To minimize the disgrace, some individuals with disabilities try to conceal their incapacity, and pretend that they comprehend what has been communicated. The interview may require extra time and patience; however, psychological preparation of the patient is crucial to accept or reject treatment.[78,79]

TREATMENT AND PREVENTION

Treatment of patients with DS follows the same principles as for the general population, with the institution of extra measures. Behavioral challenges, IQ, medications, and physical status may require some adjustments.

Most children with DS are affectionate and cooperative for dental treatment, and may only require the techniques used in treating other pediatric patients, like Tell, Show, and Do.[72,80] However, uncooperative patients may require treatment under sedation or general anesthesia in the dental office or medical facilities. Dental practitioners should refer to the patient's physician, whenever needed, to avoid any medical risk.[80]

Susceptibility to Infections

The variations from the normal immune system in individuals with DS make them more susceptible to infections. These abnormalities are T-cell and B-cell lymphopenia, diminished response to vaccinations, and neutrophil chemotaxis. Other nonimmunologic factors include zinc deficiency and anatomic variations.[81] Thus, compromised dental health may represent a risk for systemic disease, especially in patients with simultaneous medical issues. Prophylactic regimens should be implemented for any probability of risk to the patient.[67,80]

Prevention

In medically compromised individuals, institution of all possible preventive measures is needed to prevent diseases and lessen suffering.[82] Studies have shown that children with DS with limited or no prevention tend to have more teeth extracted; more decayed, missing or filled teeth; poor oral health; and unmet treatment needs.[17,83] Also, more emphasis is placed on health issues other than oral health, so parents do not receive prevention information in early childhood.[17] Prolonged bottle feeding and low salivary levels increase the risk of baby bottle syndrome among these individuals.[17] A prevention strategy should be individualized to each patient incorporating the following[17,72,82,84]:

- Early intervention and advice with parents' participation and education
- Early and regular visit to the dental office, staring at 12 to 18 months
- Scaling, prophylaxis, oral hygiene motivation, and brushing
- Topical fluoride application; 3 to 4/y
- Fissure sealants
- Reduced recall interval
- Diet and assistance in adopting good dietary practice

Oral hygiene should be performed by parents/caregivers until the patient is proficient.

Restorative

Children with DS should limit caries risk factors such as frequent sweets intake and prolonged use of a bottle. Early education of the children and parents/caregivers about prevention should be instituted.[10,72] All restorative treatments should be performed, as for normal individuals, using behavioral management techniques.[72] Some individuals with DS require sedation or general anesthesia.[72] Areas of erosion and developmental defects of dentin may require full coronal coverage rather than simple restorations.[82]

Endodontics

Pulp therapy depends on many factors: IQ, physical status, and periodontal status of the patient.[85] Pulp therapy should be avoided in children with DS with heart defects.[82] Differences in root canal anatomy among the DS population has not been fully studied. Kelsen and colleagues[86] in 1999 reported that the crown and root length of anterior and premolar teeth is shorter. Root canals are usually single with a decreased incidence of lateral canals and irregularities. A single-visit root canal therapy could be a practical option, particularly for those patients in whom general anesthesia/medications might be required, and particularly with the use of advanced dental technologies such as apex locators.[87]

Periodontal Treatment

Both surgical and nonsurgical therapies showed a comparative clinical effect. The immunologic impairment can be overwhelmed and does not interfere with proper clinical healing and maintenance.[88] Consequently, the principal issue in the management of periodontitis in patients with DS is prevention. Prevention includes all the measures specified for prevention, along with the use of medicaments as needed.[72,82] In circumstances in which vulnerability to periodontitis is encountered, an aggressive treatment should be instituted.[82,89] Individualized nonsurgical periodontal therapy is planned with suitable changes, including[84,89–94]:

- Early intervention through regular scaling and root planing in conjunction with locally delivered antiinfective agents, in addition to the use of chlorhexidine mouthwashes.
- Supervised tooth brushing program with continuous motivation.
- Continuous review program every 3 months with conventional therapy and oral hygiene reinforcement and motivation. In this way the poor plaque control may be overcome. The effectiveness of this regimen could result from supragingival plaque harboring pathogens for reinfection. Also, the maximum clinical effect is attained after 3 months and maintained until 6 months after therapy, because a single visit has no effect.[95]
- Medicaments showing comparable effects have been proposed to be used in combination with conventional therapy. Local administration of tetracycline and chlorhexidine mouthwash is reported to cause moderate attachment gain, reduction of pocket depths, and stabilization of periodontal status.
- Integration of disclosing agent in the dentifrices, and thus dental plaque observation, can produce a noticeable reduction in plaque index.
- Combination of disclosing agent such as erythrosine and chlorhexidine is best for the reduction of both plaque index and gingival bleeding. Toothpastes are an easy and acceptable method to deliver therapeutic agents.
- Low-level laser therapy has been shown to have an effect similar to antibacterial medicaments. Combination therapy with conventional methods has been shown to be effective for up to 6 weeks after treatment.

Orthodontic Intervention

Malocclusion and craniofacial characteristics of individuals with DS clearly indicate that these patients benefit from orthodontic correction and intervention. The level of mental insufficiency may have caused dental experts to be timid in dealing with the related malocclusions.[96] A person with DS may present with variety of conditions that can be corrected by orthodontic treatment/intervention; for example[96,97]:

1. Maxillary anteroposterior and horizontal hypoplasia
2. Congenitally missing and impacted teeth
3. Tooth size discrepancy
4. Anterior open bite
5. Tongue thrust and relative macroglossia
6. Anterior diastema (crowding and spacing)
7. Narrow palatal vault
8. Chewing difficulties leading to frequent choking episodes

These abnormalities may affect appearance and some vital functions, such as speaking and swallowing. Thus orthodontic intervention and correction using a 2-phase or multiphase treatment might be required. A promising result is more likely through implementing a well-coordinated interdisciplinary approach. The following has been recommended in the literature to assist in orthodontic treatment[96–99]:

1. Before commencing, decide on the level of tolerance and cooperation.
2. The use of behavioral management and psychological approaches.
3. The use of fast-setting impression materials with pleasant flavors.
4. Easy bonding of brackets.
5. The use of memory-type wires and self-ligating brackets.

6. Use of the current and advanced planning and techniques in orthognathic surgery.
7. Implant replacement of congenitally missing teeth. Usage of temporary anchorage devices.
8. Early appliance therapy using a Castillo-Morales plate to stimulate and improve orofacial musculature function. Oromotor therapy can be combined with other functional orthodontic treatments, speech therapy, and physiotherapy.

DENTAL IMPLANTS

The literature contains few case reports of successful results. Partially or completely edentulous patients with implant-supported prostheses have achieved high success rates and patient satisfaction compared with traditional techniques. The treatment should include a multidisciplinary approach to restore function, phonetics, and esthetics in these patients. Rigorous oral hygiene and motivation should be implemented for long-term results and to prevent soft tissue inflammation. Systemic conditions, macroglossia, developmental anomalies of teeth, bone quality, and cooperation may influence or interfere with implant placement.[100–102]

Prosthetic Treatment

In general, patients with DS do not favor removable dentures. In contrast, prosthetic techniques may present difficulties in patients with DS. The use of sectional impression procedures and a McKesson mouth prop to keep the mouth open is effective. A fast-setting impression material should be used, with care taken to avoid the impression material entering the pharynx or remaining in the mouth.[103]

GAG REFLEX

The gag reflex is more prominent in patients with DS. This reflex can be evoked even in the anterior area. Consequently, dental examination of the posterior area may induce gaging and possibly gastroesophageal reflux. The reflux is normally uncomfortable and results in a refusal of further treatment. The gag reflex may be reduced by behavioral modifications such as relaxation and distraction. It can be also lessened by the use of facial and intraoral massage, and pharmacologic or nonpharmacologic interventions.[67,104]

General Anesthesia Management

General anesthesia can be used for the treatment of some patients with DS, but it is crucial to recognize differences between patients and their implications. For example, airway anomalies, endocrine disorders, and congenital heart disorders may require some modifications or consideration for general anesthesia. These patients are also more prone to hypothermia during surgery or to developing spinal cord damage from atlantoaxial subluxation. Preoperative and postoperative morbidities are also more common.[82,105]

TOOTH WEAR AND BRUXISM

High levels of tooth wear (attrition and erosion) among persons with DS are largely caused by bruxism and an acidic oral environment (gastric reflux and vomiting). The cause of bruxism is multifactorial: anxiety, malocclusion, underdevelopment of nervous control, and laxity of the temporomandibular joint ligaments. Patients should be placed on periodic assessment to prevent/identify tooth wear. Educational programs should be implemented to increase awareness. For individuals with bruxism, dental screening of any occlusal and/or oral health abnormalities and behavioral evaluation are required. Behavioral intervention for individuals with bruxism might be required.[106] The use of an equilibrated bite raising appliance may help in cases in which occlusal adjustment is not attempted or is unrealistic.[67,107]

Dental Trauma

Walking difficulties in patients with DS make them more susceptible to dental trauma.[108] Tooth fracture or luxation, particularly in the anterior teeth, commonly compromises pulp vitality.[67,109]

SYSTEMIC CONSIDERATIONS

There are a significant number of recognized systemic anomalies in individuals with DS that can influence oral health or interfere with treatment. These anomalies are summarized here with respect to how they can influence oral health/management[72,110–115]:

- Cardiovascular problems
  - Multiple congenital cardiac defects
  - The need for antibiotic prophylaxis should be assessed
  - Risk of infective endocarditis
  - Increased general anesthesia
- Respiratory abnormalities
  - Tracheal stenosis (general anesthesia intubation)
  - Increased risk of infections and aspiration
- Endocrine problems
  - Hypothyroidism and diabetes: oral effects of disease
- Epilepsy
  - Antiepileptic drug side effects
  - Oral tissues damage caused by seizures
  - Drug interaction
  - Identify the risk of seizures
- Gastrointestinal problems
  - Esophageal reflux and vomiting (erosions)
- Hematological problems
  - Increased risk of leukemia (10-fold to 20-fold)
- Immunologic abnormalities
  - Risk of infections
  - Increased prevalence of oral diseases such as periodontitis
- Neurologic problems
  - Deficit in motor skills and executive functions
  - Limited coordination (tends to improve with age)
  - Atypical language processing and organization
- Obstructive sleep apnea
  - Predisposing factors are anatomic: enlarged adenoid and lingual tonsils
  - If untreated, can cause pulmonary hypotension and congestive heart failure
  - Construction of oral appliances, such as mandibular advancement devices
- Skeletal problems
  - Atlantoaxial instability: maintain the neck in neutral position and use soft collar, particularly during and after general anesthesia (GA)
- Visual problems
  - Ocular disorders, such as cataract and epiphora
- Auditory problems
  - Hearing loss

REFERENCES

1. Desai SS. Down syndrome: a review of the literature. Oral Surg Oral Med Oral Pathol Oral Radiol Endod 1997;84(3):279–85.
2. Ellis H. John Langdon Down: Down's syndrome. J Perioper Pract 2013;23(12): 296–7. Available at: MEDLINE Complete, Ipswich, MA.
3. Allt J, Howell C. Down's syndrome. British Journal of Anaesthesia 2003;3(3):83–6.
4. Hultén MA, Patel SD, Tankimanova M, et al. On the origin of trisomy 21 Down syndrome. Mol Cytogenet 2008;1:21.
5. El-Gilany A-H, Yahia S, Shoker M, et al. Cytogenetic and comorbidity profile of Down syndrome in Mansoura University Children's Hospital, Egypt. Indian J Hum Genet 2011;17(3):157–63.
6. Flores-Ramírez F, Palacios-Guerrero C, Morán-Barroso V, et al. Cytogenetic profile in 1,921 cases of trisomy 21 syndrome. Arch Med Res 2015;46:484–9.
7. Kolgeci S, Kolgeci J, Azemi M, et al. Cytogenetic study in children with Down syndrome among Kosova Albanian population between 2000 and 2010. Materia Sociomed 2013;25(2):131–5.
8. Stabholz A, Mann J, Sela M, et al. Caries experience, periodontal treatment needs, salivary pH, and *Streptococcus mutans* counts in a preadolescent Down syndrome population. Spec Care Dentist 1991;11(5):203–8.
9. Fung K, Allison P. A comparison of caries rates in non-institutionalized individuals with and without Down syndrome. Spec Care Dentist 2005;25(6):302–10.
10. Liu H, Chen C, Huang S, et al. The impact of dietary and tooth-brushing habits to dental caries of special school children with disability. Res Dev Disabil 2010; 31(6):1160–9.
11. Castilho A, Marta S. Evaluation of the incidence of dental caries in patients with Down syndrome after their insertion in a preventive program [in Portuguese]. Cien Saude Colet 2010;15(Suppl 2):3249–53.
12. Fung K, Lawrence H, Allison P. A paired analysis of correlates of dental restorative care in siblings with and without Down syndrome. Spec Care Dentist 2008; 28(3):85–91.
13. Deps T, Angelo G, Martins C, et al. Association between dental caries and Down Syndrome: a systematic review and meta-analysis. PLoS One 2015;10(6): e0127484.
14. Normastura AR, Norhayani Z, Azizah Y, et al. Saliva and dental caries in Down syndrome children. Sains Malays 2013;42(1):59–63.
15. Areias C, Sampaio-Maia B, Macho V, et al. Does the chemistry in the saliva of Down syndrome children explain their low caries prevalence? Eur J Paediatr Dent 2013;14(1):23–6.
16. Singh V, Arora R, Bhayya D, et al. Comparison of relationship between salivary electrolyte levels and dental caries in children with Down syndrome. J Nat Sci Biol Med 2015;6(1):144–8.
17. Shore S, Lightfoot T, Ansell P. Oral disease in children with Down syndrome: causes and prevention. Community Pract 2010;83(2):18.
18. König K. Dental morphology in relation to caries resistance with special reference to fissures as susceptible areas. J Dent Res 1963;42(1):461.
19. Singh A. Dental Caries Rates in Children with Down Syndrome. Diss. University of Illinois at Chicago, 2014. Available at: http://indigo.uic.edu/bitstream/handle/10027/19022/Singh_Amarjot.pdf?sequence=1. Accessed Febraury 06, 2015.
20. Al-Khadra T. Prevalence of dental caries and oral hygiene status among down's syndrome patients in Riyadh – Saudi Arabia. Pakistan Oral Dental J 2011;31(1):113.

21. Jain M, Mathur A, Kulkarni S, et al. Oral health status of mentally disabled subjects in India. J Oral Sci 2009;51(3):333–40.

22. Chaushu S, Yefe Nof E, Becker A, et al. Parotid salivary immunoglobulins, recurrent respiratory tract infections and gingival health in institutionalized and non-institutionalized subjects with Down's syndrome. J Intellect Disabil Res 2003; 47(2):101–7.

23. Kumar S, Sharma J, Duraiswamy P, et al. Determinants for oral hygiene and periodontal status among mentally disabled children and adolescents. J Indian Soc Pedod Prev Dent 2009;27(3):151–7.

24. Al Habashneh R, Al-Jundi S, Khader Y, et al. Oral health status and reasons for not attending dental care among 12-to 16-year-old children with Down syndrome in special needs centres in Jordan. Int J Dental Hyg 2012;10(4):259–64.

25. Ulseth J, Hestnes A, Stovner L, et al. Dental caries and periodontitis in persons with Down syndrome. Spec Care Dentist 1991;11(2):71–3.

26. Krishnan C, Archana A. Evaluation of oral hygiene status and periodontal health in mentally retarded subjects with or without Down's syndrome in comparison with normal healthy individuals. J Oral Health Community Dent 2014;8(2):91.

27. Gabre P, Martinsson T, Gahnberg L. Longitudinal study of dental caries, tooth mortality and interproximal bone loss in adults with intellectual disability. Eur J Oral Sci 2001;109(1):20–6.

28. Amano A, Murakami J, Akiyama S, et al. Review article: etiologic factors of early-onset periodontal disease in Down syndrome. Jpn Dent Sci Rev 2008;44: 118–27.

29. Ahmed N, Parthasarathy H, Arshad M, et al. Assessment of *Porphyromonas gingivalis* and *Aggregatibacter actinomycetemcomitans* in Down's syndrome subjects and systemically healthy subjects: A comparative clinical trial. J Indian Soc Periodontol 2014;18(6):728–33.

30. Khocht A, Yaskell T, Socransky S, et al. Subgingival microbiota in adult Down syndrome periodontitis. J Periodont Res 2012;47(4):500–7.

31. Khocht A, Russell B, Cannon J, et al. Phagocytic cell activity and periodontitis in Down syndrome. Oral Dis 2012;18(4):346.

32. Amano A, Kishima T, Morisaki I, et al. Periodontopathic bacteria in children with Down syndrome. J Periodontol 2000;71(2):249.

33. Khocht A, Russell B, Cannon J, et al. Oxidative burst intensity of peripheral phagocytic cells and periodontitis in Down syndrome. J Periodont Res 2014; 49(1):29–35.

34. Rodrigues Freire I, Coelho Ávila Aguiar S, Penha de Oliveira S. Functional activity of neutrophils and systemic inflammatory response of Down's syndrome patients with periodontal disease. Braz J Oral Sci 2012;11(3):422.

35. López-Pérez R, Borges-Yáñez S, Jiménez-García G, et al. Oral hygiene, gingivitis, and periodontitis in persons with Down syndrome. Spec Care Dentist 2002;22(6): 214–20.

36. Tsilingaridis G, Yucel-Lindberg T, Concha Quezada H, et al. The relationship between matrix metalloproteinases (MMP-3, -8, -9) in serum and peripheral lymphocytes (CD8+, CD56+) in Down syndrome children with gingivitis. J Periodont Res 2014;49(6):742.

37. Al-Sufyani G, Al-Maweri S, Al-Ghashm A, et al. Oral hygiene and gingival health status of children with Down syndrome in Yemen: a cross-sectional study. J Int Soc Prev Community Dent 2014;4(2):82–6.

38. Zizzi A, Piemontese M, Aspriello S, et al. Periodontal status in the Down's syndrome subjects living in central-eastern Italy: the effects of place of living. Int J Dental Hyg 2014;12(3):193–8.
39. Solanki J, Gupta S, Arya A. Dental caries and periodontal status of mentally handicapped institutilized children. J Clin Diagn Res 2014;8(7):25–7.
40. Morinushi T, Lopatin D, Nakao R, et al. A comparison of the gingival health of children with Down syndrome to healthy children residing in an institution. Spec Care Dentist 2006;26(1):13–9.
41. Khocht A, Janal M, Turner B. Periodontal health in Down syndrome: contributions of mental disability, personal, and professional dental care. Spec Care Dentist 2010;30(3):118–23.
42. De Castilho ARF, Pardi V, Pereira CV. Caries prevalence, level of mutans streptococci, salivary flow rate, and buffering capacity in subjects with Down syndrome. Braz J Oral Sci 2007;21(6):1331–6.
43. Moreira M, Schwertner C, Grando D, et al. Oral health status and salivary levels of mutans streptococci in children with Down syndrome. Pediatr Dent 2015; 37(4):355–60.
44. Castilho A, Pardi V, Pereira C. Dental caries experience in relation to salivary findings and molecular identification of S. mutans and S. sobrinus in subjects with Down syndrome. Odontology 2011;99(2):162.
45. Cogulu D, Sabah E, Kutukculer N, et al. Evaluation of the relationship between caries indices and salivary secretory IgA, salivary pH, buffering capacity and flow rate in children with Down's syndrome. Arch Oral Biol 2006;51:23–8.
46. Ahmadi-Motamayel F, Goodarzi M, Hendi S, et al. Total antioxidant capacity of saliva and dental caries. Med Oral Patol Oral Cir Bucal 2013;18(4):e553–6.
47. Levine M, Herzberg M, van Dyke T, et al. Specificity of salivary-bacterial interactions: role of terminal sialic acid residues in the interaction of salivary glycoproteins with Streptococcus sanguis and Streptococcus mutans. Infect Immun 1978;19(1): 107–15.
48. Arki A, Gagneux P. Multifarious roles of sialic acids in immunity. Ann N Y Acad Sci 2012;1253:16–36.
49. Subramaniam P, Girish Babu K, Mohan Das L. Assessment of salivary total antioxidant levels and oral health status in children with Down syndrome. Spec Care Dentist 2014;34(4):193.
50. Bogdan C. Nitric oxide and the immune response. Nat Immunol 2001;2:907–16.
51. de Sousa M, Vieira R, de Oliveira L, et al. Antioxidants and biomarkers of oxidative damage in the saliva of patients with Down's syndrome. Arch Oral Biol 2015; 60:600–5.
52. Davidovich E, Aframian D, Shapira J, et al. A comparison of the sialochemistry, oral pH, and oral health status of down syndrome children to healthy children. Int J Paediatr Dent 2010;20(4):235.
53. Macho V, Coelho A, Areias C, et al. Craniofacial features and specific oral characteristics of Down syndrome children. Oral Health Dent Manag 2014;13(2):408–11.
54. Vigild M. Prevalence of malocclusion in mentally retarded young adults. Community Dent Oral Epidemiol 1985;13(3):183.
55. Macho V, Andrade D, Areias C, et al. Comparative study of the prevalence of occlusal anomalies in Down Syndrome children and their siblings. Br J Med Res 2014;4(35):5604–11.
56. Rahim F, Mohamed A, Nor M, et al. Malocclusion and orthodontic treatment need evaluated among subjects with Down syndrome using the Dental Aesthetic Index (DAI). Angle Orthod 2014;84(4):600–6.

57. Meštrović S, Mikšić M, Štefanac-Papić J, et al. Prevalence of malocclusion in patients with Down's syndrome. Acta Stomatol Croat 2002;36(2):239–41.
58. Mari Eli Leonelli de M, Luiz Cesar de M, Gustavo Nogara D, et al. Dental anomalies in patients with down syndrome. Braz Dent J 2007;18(4):346.
59. Shapira J, Chaushu S, Becker A. Prevalence of tooth transposition, third molar agenesis, and maxillary canine impaction in individuals with Down syndrome. Angle Orthod 2000;70(4):290–6.
60. Shukla D, Bablani D, Chowdhry A, et al. Dentofacial and cranial changes in Down syndrome [Original article]. Osong Public Health Res Perspect 2014;5:339–44.
61. Acerbi A, de Freitas C, de Magalhães M. Prevalence of numeric anomalies in the permanent dentition of patients with Down syndrome. Spec Care Dentist 2001;21(2):75–8.
62. Ghaib NH, Al-Khatieeb MM, Abd Awn DH. Hypodontia in Downs syndrome patients. J Bagh Coll Dentistry 2009;21(No 1):98–103.
63. Jaspers MT. Taurodontism in the Down syndrome. Oral Surg Oral Med Oral Pathol 1981;51(6):632–6.
64. Bell J, Civil C, Townsend G, et al. The prevalence of taurodontism in Down's syndrome. J Ment Defic Res 1989;33(6):467–76.
65. Frostad WA, Cleall JF, Melosky LC. Craniofacial complex in the trisomy 21 syndrome (Down's syndrome). Arch Oral Biol 1971;16(7):707–22.
66. Suri S, Tompson B, Cornfoot L. Cranial base, maxillary and mandibular morphology in Down syndrome. Angle Orthod 2010;80(5):861–9.
67. Hennequin M, Faulks D, Veyrune J, et al. Significance of oral health in persons with Down syndrome: a literature review. Dev Med Child Neurol 1999;41(4):275–83.
68. Asokan S, Muthu MS, Sivakumar N. Oral findings of Down syndrome children in Chennai city, India. Indian J Dent Res 2008;19:230–5.
69. Schendel S, Gorlin R. Frequency of cleft uvula and submucous cleft palate in patients with Down's syndrome. J Dent Res 1974;53(4):840.
70. Rigoldi C, Galli M, Albertini G, et al. Gait strategy in patients with Ehlers-Danlos syndrome hypermobility type and Down syndrome. Res Dev Disabil 2012;33:1437–42.
71. Odeh M, Hershkovits M, Bornstein J, et al. Congenital absence of salivary glands in Down syndrome. Arch Dis Child 2013;98(10):781–3.
72. Cheng RHW, Yiu CKY, Keung Leung W. Oral Health in Individuals with Down Syndrome. In: Dey S, editor. Prenatal Diagnosis and Screening for Down Syndrome. INTECH Open Access Publisher; 2011. Available at: http://www.intechopen.com/books/prenatal-diagnosis-and-screening-for-down-syndrome/oral-health-in-individuals-with-down-syndrome.
73. Rahim F, Mohamed A, Nor M, et al. Dental care access among individuals with Down syndrome: a Malaysian scenario. Acta Odontol Scand 2014;72(8):999–1004.
74. Allison P, Hennequin M, Faulks D. Dental care access among individuals with Down syndrome in France. Spec Care Dentist 2000;20(1):28–34.
75. Roberts JE, Price J, Malkin C. Language and communication development in Down syndrome. Ment Retard Dev Disabil Res Rev 2007;13(1):26–35.
76. Buckley SJ. Speech, language and communication for individuals with Down syndrome — An overview. Down syndrome issues and information. 2000. http://www.down-syndrome.org/information/language/overview/. Accessed September 29, 2015.
77. Dougall A, Fiske J. Access to spec care dentist, part 2. Commun Br Dental J 2008;205(1):11–21.

78. Tassé MJ, Schalock R, Thompson JR, et al. Guidelines for interviewing people with disabilities: supports intensity scale. Washington, DC: American Association on Intellectual and Developmental Disabilities; 2005.
79. Smith DS. Health care management of adults with Down syndrome. Am Fam Physician 2001;64(6):1031–44.
80. Jeng W, Wang T, Cher T, et al. Strategies for oral health care for people with disabilities in Taiwan. J Dent Sci 2009;4(4):165–72.
81. Ram G, Chinen J. Infections and immunodeficiency in Down syndrome. Clin Exp Immunol 2011;164(1):9–16.
82. Prakash A, Raghuwanshi B, Hameed A. Down syndrome- diagnosis and guidelines of dental and orthodontic management. Guident 2013;6(4):40–2.
83. Sari M, Ozmen B, Koyuturk A, et al. A retrospective comparison of dental treatment under general anesthesia on children with and without mental disabilities. Niger J Clin Pract 2014;17(3):361–5.
84. Sakellari D, Belibasakis G, Chadjipadelis T, et al. Supragingival and subgingival microbiota of adult patients with Down's syndrome. Changes after periodontal treatment. Oral Microbiol Immunol 2001;16(6):376–82.
85. Gulabivala K, Ng Y. Endodontics. 4th edition. Elsevier, Mosby; 2014. p. 366. (Chapter 15).
86. Kelsen A, Love R, Kieser J, et al. Root canal anatomy of anterior and premolar teeth in Down's syndrome. Int Endod J 1999;32(3):211–6.
87. Yap E, Parashos P, Borromeo G. Root canal treatment and special needs patients. Int Endod J 2015;48(4):351.
88. Zaldivar-Chiapa R, Arce-Mendoza A, Rosa-Ramirez M, et al. Evaluation of surgical and non-surgical periodontal therapies, and immunological status, of young Down's syndrome patients. J Periodontol 2005;76(7):1061–5.
89. Gautami P, Ramaraju A, Gunashekhar M. Adjunctive use of tetracycline fibers with nonsurgical periodontal therapy in an adult with Down syndrome: a case report. Spec Care Dentist 2012;32(2):61–5.
90. Yoshihara T, Morinushi T, Kinjyo S, et al. Effect of periodic preventive care on the progression of periodontal disease in young adults with Down's syndrome. J Clin Periodontol 2005;32(6):556–60.
91. Shyama M, Al-Mutawa S, Honkala S, et al. Supervised toothbrushing and oral health education program in Kuwait for children and young adults with Down syndrome. Spec Care Dentist 2003;23(3):94–9.
92. Teitelbaum A, Pochapski M, Jansen J, et al. Evaluation of the mechanical and chemical control of dental biofilm in patients with Down syndrome. Community Dent Oral Epidemiol 2009;37(5):463.
93. ElShenawy H, Elkhodary A, Saafan A, et al. Management of periodontitis in patients with Down syndrome using low energy diode laser. WebmedCentral DENTISTRY 2010;1(10):WMC00990. http://dx.doi.org/10.9754/journal.wmc.2010.00990.
94. Sharaf H, Elkhodary A, Saafan A, et al. Antibacterial effectiveness of low energy diode laser irradiation on management of periodontitis in Down syndrome. Egypt J Hosp Med 2012;47:226.
95. Zigmond M, Stabholz A, Chaushu S, et al. The outcome of a preventive dental care programme on the prevalence of localized aggressive periodontitis in Down's syndrome individuals. J Intellect Disabil Res 2006;50(7):492–500.
96. Rao D, Hegde S, Naik S, et al. Malocclusion in down syndrome - a review. S Afr Dent J 2015;(1):12–5.
97. Musich DR. Orthodontic intervention and patients with down syndrome: the role of inclusion, technology and leadership. Angle Orthod 2006;76(4):734–5.

98. Marques LS, Alcântara CE, Pereira LJ, et al. Down syndrome: a risk factor for malocclusion severity? Braz Oral Res 2015;29:44.

99. Giese R. Retrospective clinical investigation of the impact of early treatment of children with Down's syndrome according to Castillo-Morales. J Orofac Orthop 2001;62(4):255.

100. Ribeiro C, Siqueira A, Bez L, et al. Dental implant rehabilitation of a patient with Down syndrome: a case report. J Oral Implantol 2011;37(4):481–7.

101. Bergendal B, Nilsson P, Olson L. Dental implants in a patient with Down's syndrome. IADH, International Association of Disability and Oral Health, Aten, Grekland, 2002. Odontologisk Riksstämma, Göteborg, 2002. Swed Dent J 2002;26:183–4.

102. Lustig JP, Yanko R, Zilberman U. Use of dental implants in patients with Down syndrome: a case report. Spec Care Dentist 2002;22(5):201–4.

103. Scully C. Down's syndrome: aspects of dental care. J Dent 1976;4(4):167–74.

104. Abanto J, Ciamponi A, Francischini E, et al. Medical problems and oral care of patients with Down syndrome: a literature review. Spec Care Dentist 2011;31(6):197–203.

105. Meitzner M, Skurnowicz J. Anesthetic considerations for patients with Down syndrome. AANA J 2005;73(2):103–7.

106. Lang R, White P, Didden R, et al. Review: treatment of bruxism in individuals with developmental disabilities: a systematic review. Res Dev Disabil 2009;30:809–18.

107. Bell E, Kaidonis J, Townsend G. Tooth wear in children with Down syndrome. Aust Dent J 2002;47(1):30–5.

108. Galli M, Cimolin V, Rigoldi C, et al. The effects of low arched feet on foot rotation during gait in children with Down syndrome. J Intellect Disabil Res 2014;58(8):758–64.

109. Mônica Regina Pereira Senra S, Fernanda Oliveira de P, Maria das Graças Afonso Miranda C, et al. Patient with Down syndrome and implant therapy: a case report. Braz Dent J 2010;21(6):550–4. Available at: http://www.scielo.br/scielo.php?script=sci_arttext&pid=S0103-64402010000600012&lng=en.

110. Schott N, Holfelder B. Relationship between motor skill competency and executive function in children with Down's syndrome. J Intellect Disabil Res 2015;59(9):860–72 (17991).

111. Jacola L, Byars A, Hickey F, et al. Functional magnetic resonance imaging of story listening in adolescents and young adults with Down syndrome: evidence for atypical neurodevelopment. J Intellect Disabil Res 2014;58(10):892–902.

112. Prasher V. Down syndrome and thyroid disorders: a review. Downs Syndr Res Pract 1999;6(1):25–42.

113. Stephen E, Dickson J, Kindley AD, et al. Surveillance of vision and ocular disorders in children with Down syndrome. Dev Med Child Neurol 2007;49(7):513–5.

114. Agarwal Gupta N, Kabra M. Diagnosis and management of Down syndrome. Indian J Pediatr 2014;81(6):560–7.

115. Aragon CE, Burneo JG. Understanding the patient with epilepsy and seizures in the dental practice. J Can Dent Assoc 2007;73(1):71–6.

Americans with Disabilities Act

Its Importance in Special Care Dentistry

Stanley R. Surabian, DDS, JD, FACD, FICD, DABSCD

KEYWORDS

- Special care dentistry • Americans with Disabilities Act
- *Diagnostic and Statistical Manual of Mental Disorders* (Fifth Edition)
- Developmental disabilities • Intellectual disability • Autism spectrum disorder
- Epilepsy • Cerebral palsy

KEY POINTS

- This article focuses on understanding the Americans with Disabilities Act (AwDA) and developmental disabilities for health care providers in special care dentistry. Essential to this awareness is a comprehension of statutory and regulatory requirements, in particular the federal ADA, and how state disability acts can be even more rigorous in their application.
- Developmental disabilities are re-examined in the context of the *Diagnostic and Statistical Manual of Mental Disorders* (Fifth Edition) (*DSM-5*), including updated terminology and definitions.
- Understanding of intellectual disability, epilepsy, autism spectrum disorder (ASD), and cerebral palsy is necessary because the management of oral health considerations for special care patients has become ever more complex and indispensable.

For one Long Island, New York, father, an issue that has been building for 2 years appears to be headed to a dramatic head on his son's first day of school. Christian Killoran of Remsenburg, New York, wants his 12-year-old son, who has Down syndrome, to attend the same middle school as his friends and siblings, but says the Westhampton Beach School District will not let Aiden Killoran in. But his dad says he plans to show up at the school on the first day, Wednesday, with Aiden and supporters. The school had requested a temporary restraining order to keep the Killorans off school property. In U.S. District Court on Monday, the family and the school reached an agreement that a restraining order would not be needed. "They [the Westhampton School District] has never in history allowed an alternately assessed special education student to attend its middle school," Killoran told ABC News of students with disabilities whose performance is evaluated

Community Regional Medical Center, Surabian Dental Care Center, 290 North Wayte Lane, 2500, Fresno, CA 93701, USA
E-mail address: ssurabiandds@communitymedical.org

Dent Clin N Am 60 (2016) 627–647
http://dx.doi.org/10.1016/j.cden.2016.02.008 **dental.theclinics.com**
0011-8532/16/$ – see front matter © 2016 Elsevier Inc. All rights reserved.

in ways other than traditional testing. These would include students with cognitive and other disabilities. Killoran said denying Aiden entry is a violation of his civil rights... "We told them 2 years ago we would not be victimized by their culture [of not allowing certain students with special needs entry] and wanted to develop a plan," Killoran said. Professor Sue Buckley, director for Science and Research at Down Syndrome Education International in Portsmouth, U.K., said in an email to ABC News, "I am appalled and saddened that any school should prevent a father and child from entering the grounds by law. All the research studies show children with Down syndrome achieve more in inclusive education—better reading, maths and spoken language outcomes, more socially mature and fewer behavior challenges—yet many US school districts seem to ignore this information. All children should be welcomed in their local community. What message are the educators giving all the other children in their school if they exclude a child with Down syndrome? I agree this is a clear case of disability discrimination," added Buckley, a leading expert on inclusion for students with Down syndrome. ... But Killoran said Aiden has a right to attend the same school as the kids he has known all his life and not be discriminated against because of his diagnosis. Aiden, who he called "incredible" is the first student with Down syndrome to graduate from Remsenburg-Speonk elementary. "If you ask the community what they want, you'd find they also want Aiden included. Everyone benefits from his empathy and kindness. We have faith in the school, teacher and staff to provide him with a great education and are committed to changing this."[1]

In 2000, the US Department of Health and Human Services published *Oral Health in America: A Report of the Surgeon General*. The report stated the scope of the problem related to those individuals defined as disabled under the AwDA:

The oral health problems of individuals with disabilities are complex. These problems may be due to underlying congenital anomalies as well as to inability to receive the personal and professional health care needed to maintain oral health. There are more than 54 million individuals defined as disabled under the Americans with Disabilities Act, including almost a million children under age 6 and 4.5 million children between 6 and 16 years of age.[2]

The report offered its conclusion that known barriers between people seeking oral health services and the provision of oral health services should be eliminated:

Individuals whose health is physically, mentally and emotionally compromised need comprehensive integrated care. ... Given the wide variability among groups with disabilities...more in-depth assessment and analysis of the determinants of oral health status, access to care and the role of health in the overall quality of life and life expectancy is needed.[2]

This article looks at various approaches to define the word, *disability*. No one idea defines the word; however, its use is inclusionary, particularly as defined in the AwDA. A developmental disability is regarded differently from a sprained ankle. A developmental disability is well defined under law and common use as a broad category coming within the AwDA. Dentists need to be aware of the different permutations of the use of the term. Although a broken femur may qualify as a disability under health and disability insurance, it may not be a disability within the scope of the AwDA.

The first broad area of discussion is the AwDA, from definitions and discussion through disability access claims. The second broad area of discussion is to ascribe meaning to the term, *developmental disability*. For dental health professionals, in particular those caring for patients with special care needs, it is essential to have an understanding of the use of these terms to understand the conditions that often present in practice.

AMERICANS WITH DISABILITIES ACT

The AwDA was enacted into law on July 26, 1990. On January 26, 1992, dental offices were added to the ADA as "places of public accommodation," requiring that the dentists serve persons qualifying as disabled under the ADA.[3-5] Discrimination is prohibited in access to service and employment for those who qualify. The federal definition of an AwDA-qualified impairment has several components.

1. The term disability means, with respect to an individual, having 1 of the following:
   a. A physical or mental impairment that substantially limits 1 or more of major life activities of such individual
   b. A record of such an impairment
   c. Being regarded as having such impairment
2. Major life activities
   a. In general, for purposes of paragraph (1), major life activities include, but are not limited to, caring for oneself, performing manual tasks, seeing, hearing, eating, sleeping, walking, standing, lifting, bending, speaking, breathing, learning, reading, concentrating, thinking, communicating, and working.
   b. Major bodily functions: for purposes of paragraph (1), a major life activity also includes the operation of a major bodily function, including but not limited to, functions of the immune system, normal cell growth, and digestive, bowel, bladder, neurologic, brain, respiratory, circulatory, endocrine, and reproductive functions.
3. Regarded as having such an impairment: for purposes of paragraph (1) (C):
   a. An individual meets the requirement of "being regarded as having such an impairment" if the individual establishes that he or she has been subjected to an action prohibited under the ADA because of an actual or perceived physical or mental impairment, whether or not the impairment limits or is perceived to limit a major life activity.
   b. Paragraph (1) (C) shall not apply to impairments that are transitory and minor. A transitory impairment is an impairment with an actual or expected duration of 6 months or less.[3]

The federal AwDA definition uses the term, *substantially limits*, whereas, for example, the State of California definition uses the term, *limits*. The term, limits, is generally a more broadly defined term; so, states using limits instead of the federal term, substantially limits, are more expansive in scope in defining an AwDA disability. The use of the federal term, substantially limits, must be understood in the context of federal acts and regulations. The US Equal Employment Opportunity Commission (EEOC) is the agency responsible for developing and implementing AwDA regulation. The AwDA Amendments Act of 2008 (ADAAA) was enacted in 2008 and published in the *Federal Register* on March 25, 2011.[6] Congress believed that court interpretations had too narrowly construed the definition of disability. As a result, many individuals with cancer, diabetes, and even a developmental disability, such as epilepsy, were denied protection under the AwDA. Congress based its decision on a declared set of findings. These findings were the basis for amendments found in the ADAAA in Section 2(a)[3]:

1. In enacting the ADA, Congress intended that the ADA "provide a clear and comprehensive national mandate for the elimination of discrimination against individuals with disabilities" and provide broad coverage.

2. In enacting the ADA, Congress recognized that physical and mental disabilities in no way diminish a person's right to fully participate in all aspects of society but that people with physical or mental disabilities are frequently precluded from doing so because of prejudice, antiquated attitudes, or the failure to remove societal and institutional barriers.

3. Although Congress expected that the definition of disability under the ADA would be interpreted consistently with how courts had applied the definition of a handicapped individual under the Rehabilitation Act of 1973, that expectation has not been fulfilled.

4. The holdings of the Supreme Court in *Sutton v. United Air Lines, Inc*, 527 U.S. 471 (1999), and its companion cases have narrowed the broad scope of protection intended to be afforded by the ADA, thus eliminating protection for many individuals whom Congress intended to protect.

5. The holding of the Supreme Court in *Toyota Motor Manufacturing, Kentucky, Inc v. Williams*, 534 U.S. 184 (2002), further narrowed the broad scope of protection intended to be afforded by the ADA.

6. As a result of these Supreme Court cases, lower courts have incorrectly found in individual cases that people with a range of substantially limiting impairments are not people with disabilities.

7. In particular, the Supreme Court, in the case of *Toyota Motor Manufacturing, Kentucky, Inc v. Williams*, 534 U.S. 184 (2002), interpreted the term, substantially limits, to require a greater degree of limitation than intended by Congress.

8. Congress finds that the current EEOC ADA regulations defining the term, substantially limits, as "significantly restricted" are inconsistent with congressional intent, by expressing too high a standard.

Congress then mandated that EEOC broadly construe new regulations of the definition of "disability." The rules of construction are to determine if an individual is substantially limited in performing a major life activity. The term, substantially limits, requires the following interpretation[6]:

- A lower degree of functional limitation than previously applied by the courts can be a substantial limitation. Although not every impairment can be defined as a disability, it does not require a significant impairment to substantially limit a major life activity.
- The term must be broadly construed in favor of maximum coverage.
- A substantial limitation of a major life activity still requires an individual assessment.
- The determination of whether an impairment of a major life activity must be made without regard to mitigating measures, such as medications, with one exception (ordinary glasses or contact lenses).
- An episodic impairment or in remission remains a disability, if, when active, it substantially limits a major activity.
- The determination of whether discrimination occurred should not require extensive analysis.
- The focus for establishing coverage is based on how an individual has been treated because of the impairment rather than the employer's belief.
- To qualify for a reasonable accommodation, an individual must be covered as having an "actual disability" or a "record of disability."

Attorney Emily Benfer gives 4 examples of the term, substantially limits, that expand the term to include "major bodily functions." She states, "The following examples demonstrate how individuals who are substantially limited in the operation of various bodily functions qualify as disabled under the ADAAA:

- An individual with cerebral palsy is disabled because cerebral palsy substantially limits the neurological function. The individual does not need to show any further limitation under the ADAAA.
- An individual with breast cancer is disabled because in its active state, her breast cancer substantially limits the normal cell growth function.
- An individual with Hepatitis B is disabled because Hepatitis B substantially limits the digestive and liver functions...An individual need only be limited in one major bodily function to qualify as disabled.
- An individual with HIV/AIDS is disabled because the virus substantially limits the immune function."[7]

LOCAL GOVERNMENT MUST MEET THE REQUIREMENTS OF THE AMERICANS WITH DISABILITY ACT

One goal of the AwDA is to allow individuals to fully participate in community activities. To do this, municipal governments are required to follow the requirements of the AwDA. AwDA title II requires state and local governments to provide accessibility to programs and services to individuals with disabilities. Municipalities are required to do a self-evaluation to locate the facilities, programs, and services needing relocation or modification for compliance.[8]

According to the US Department of Justice, there are several problems related to mistaken beliefs by local government.

Local governments often presume they are exempt from the AwDA based on incorrect assumptions. These examples are incorrect common assumptions:

- There is no grandfather clause exemption in title II.
- There is no exemption because the municipality is small in size.

All local government must "ensure that all of their programs, services and activities, when viewed in their entirety, are accessible to people with disabilities. Program access is intended to remove physical barriers to city services, programs and activities but it does not require that a city government make each facility, or each part of a facility, accessible. For example, each restroom in a facility need not be made accessible. However, signage directing people with disabilities to the accessible features and spaces in a facility should be provided. ... City governments may choose to make structural changes to existing facilities to achieve access. ... all newly constructed city facilities must be fully accessible to people with disabilities."[8]

Curb Ramps

Individuals with mobility problems may be prohibited from access to sidewalks if there are only curbs without sloping curb ramps. Often sidewalks are modified or altered or new sidewalks are built. At those times, curb ramps must be installed.[9] These modifications allow individuals who rely on wheelchairs, scooters, and other mobility assists to gain access to sidewalks and intersection crossings and provide no detriment to fully mobile individuals.

Communication

It is a title II requirement that local governments must provide communication for persons with communication disorders. One example is an individual who is deaf or hearing impaired. For these people, a sign language interpreter may meet the need.

Supplying written materials, listening devices or systems, or large print or brailled materials is an alternative, which allows individuals with disabilities to be in the communication loop with those without these communication impairments.[8]

Ordinances

Local governments must often consider reasonable modifications to existing neutral ordinances, if these ordinances do not allow persons with mobility problems to gain access to city services. Some of these modifications may include curb ramps conflicting with setback regulations to provide a ramp to a building entrance. Persons with visual impairments may need a service dog for assist. It is logical that such a dog must be allowed into health facilities and businesses or the persons cannot gain access to necessary services.[9] Yet, there may be ordinances preventing animals to be in these facilities, which require modification to meet the mandates of the AwDA.

Supreme Court Cases

The United States Supreme Court has reviewed several cases involving interpretation of the AwDA. Two of these cases are presented to show how the law was applied in different situations:

- In *Bragdon,* the issue presented was whether an individual with asymptomatic HIV comes within the AwDA's definition of disability. The Supreme Court held that asymptomatic HIV is a physical impairment limiting a major life activity. The Supreme Court believed that although asymptomatic, the diagnosis of HIV could "substantially limit" a major bodily function, such as reproduction.[10]
- In *Olmstead*, the issue presented was whether a state-institutionalized patient was required to be moved to a community setting if the treatment professionals believe it is appropriate. The Supreme Court held that undue institutionalization qualifies as discrimination by reason of disability.[11] Based on the decision, community-based settings can eliminate unjustified institutional placement, and the move of institutionalized patients to community settings has increased since this decision was reached.

DISABILITY ACCESS CLAIMS

A concern of many health professionals, including dentists, is whether their practice offices come under the AwDA. Dental offices are considered places of public accommodation and come under the AwDA. Congressional language defines public accommodations:

The following private entities are considered public accommodations for purposes of this subchapter, if the operations affect commerce: laundromat, dry cleaner, bank, barber shop, beauty shop, travel service, shoe repair service, funeral parlor, gas station, office of an accountant or lawyer, pharmacy, insurance office, professional office of a health care provider, hospital, or other service establishment.[12]

As a result, if it is found that the office is non-AwDA compliant, then the person discriminated against can file a lawsuit against the entity. Federal regulations enforce these provisions in the regulation, which states the following:

The purpose of this part is to implement Title III of the Americans with Disabilities Act of 1990 which prohibits discrimination on the basis of disability by public accommodations and requires places of public accommodation and commercial facilities to be designed, constructed, and altered in compliance with the accessibility standards established by this part.[13,14]

A settlement agreement between the US Department of Justice and the University of Medicine and Dentistry of New Jersey (UMDNJ) was reached regarding an AwDA lawsuit in a title II action against UMDNJ. A medical student applicant was notified that he was accepted into the medical school. When he submitted health records, UMDNJ discovered that the applicant had hepatitis B and his admission was rescinded. To avoid litigation, the parties volunteered to resolve the dispute without litigation. The Department of Justice determined that complainants were not required to perform exposure-prone invasive procedures as a requirement to graduate and both parties agreed to a settlement allowing the applicant to enter medical school.[15]

In another case, the plaintiff, who required use of a wheelchair, claimed that the defendant restaurant failed to remove architectural barriers to access. The plaintiff prevailed in this case by proving all 3 factors of a successful AwDA claim. The defendant was liable for violating the AwDA and ordered to modify an entrance ramp and an exterior route to the premises. To prevail, the plaintiff had to show that he was disabled and that the defendant was a private entity that operates a place of public accommodation; the plaintiff was denied full and equal access to the restaurant.[16]

Attorneys Franklin and Thompson[17] outline the steps dental offices should take to reduce lawsuit risks:

- The first thing to do to prevent lawsuits is listen extra attentively to disabled patients and treat them with respect. This works because most disabled patients are not AwDA activists.
- If a patient with a disability complains, be positive and see if the problem can be addressed successfully, and solve it.
- Next, train the staff to think the same way.
- Staff should know which examination and procedure rooms are accessible and where portable accessible equipment is stored.
- Staff should understand how to properly assist patients who need transfers and lifts. They should know that not all persons with disabilities are the same—each is unique.
- Dentists and staff should first ask disabled patients if they need help before providing it, because many people who use wheelchairs for mobility consider their wheelchair to be an extension of their body.
- Remove construction-related barriers.
- Accessible medical equipment is required for dentists and other medical practitioners. The government asserts that examining a patient in a wheelchair usually is less thorough than on an examination table or examination chair and does not provide the patient "full and equal" medical services. Thus, availability of accessible medical equipment—specifically, medical and dental examination tables and chairs—is an important part of providing accessible medical care, and dentists and other medical care providers must ensure that medical equipment is not a barrier to individuals with disabilities.
- Further, to prevent claims, consider conducting an AwDA facility audit—or "compliance implementation plan." Plans should include an AwDA survey, which notes each barrier/compliance issue, the costs to remediate each compliance issue, and projected completion dates for items on the survey.[17]

DEVELOPMENTAL DISABILITIES

The federal definition for a developmental disability is found in the Developmental Disabilities Assistance and Bill of Rights Act (42 U.S.C. §6000 et seq.) and states the following:

> *The term developmental disability means a severe, chronic disability of an individual 5 years of age or older that – (a) Is attributable to mental or physical impairment or a combination of mental and physical impairments; (b) Is manifested before the individual attains age 22; (c) Is likely to continue indefinitely; (d) Results in substantial functional limitations in three or more of the following areas of major life activity (i) self care; (ii) receptive and expressed language; (iii) learning; (iv) mobility; (v) self-direction; (vi) capacity for independent living; and (vii) economic self-sufficiency; and (e) Reflects the individual's need for a combination and sequence of special, interdisciplinary, or generic services, supports, or other assistance that is of life-long or extended duration and is individually planned and coordinated, except that such term, when applied to infants and young children means individuals from birth to age 5, inclusive, who have substantial developmental delay or specific congenital or acquired conditions with a high probability of resulting in developmental disabilities if services are not provided.[18]*

HISTORICAL PERSPECTIVE

Starting with the federal definition of developmental disability, descriptive language is classified and used to construct a definition of a class of conditions affecting human beings. Historically, if some people were different from the majority, they had to be inferior in some way. Without any understanding, those persons with developmental disabilities were vulnerable to the attitudes of the time. Because these individuals were believed to be possessed by the devil or evil spirits, from 1200 AD to 1700 AD they were whipped, tortured, and burned at the stake. During this same time, an estimated tens of thousands women were executed as witches. English Elizabethan Poor Laws from 1598 to 1601 resulted in the use of the word, *handicap*. People with disabilities were ejected from hospitals and monastery shelters for the poor and were forced to beg, being given a cap in which to collect alms. This was the origin of the term, *handicap*. Many of the people with disabilities provided entertainment and endured humiliation in return for food and shelter.[19]

In 1692, witchcraft trials began in Salem Village of the Massachusetts Bay Colony. In 2 years, more than 200 persons were accused of witchcraft and 20 were executed. Often these women had some form of mental illness or disability. Even disease or bad fortune was taken as a sign of a fallen person, especially spiritually.[20] From 1800 to the 1920s, society still regarded these individuals as genetically defective and inferior and they were hidden or displayed as freaks and beggars. By the 1970s, society began to view persons with disabilities as more independent, recognizing civil rights while mainstreaming evolved.[19]

ETHICS

Ethics are the moral principles that govern a person's behavior or human conduct based on moral principles. Dr Thomas Beauchamp and Dr James Childress[21] developed 4 principles of what they called *biomedical ethics*, now often referred to as *principlism* (**Table 1**). The 4 biomedical principles are *nonmaleficence, beneficence, autonomy,* and *justice*. These principles are the bases of discussions on ethics involved in health care decision making. Most modern hospitals have a

Table 1 Principles of biomedical ethics	
Nonmaleficence	First do no harm
Beneficence	Do everything to benefit the patient
Autonomy	The patient makes the decision of what is to be done
Justice	Distributive justice, common good

From Beauchamp T, Childress J. Principles of biomedical ethics. 7th edition. New York: Oxford University Press; 2013; with permission.

multidisciplinary ethics committee and committee members can be called on by patients, their families, clergy, medical staff, or allied health personnel to offer guidance in understanding and decision making.[21,22] Each principle is defined and discussed to see how it effects understanding of disabilities.

Nonmaleficence – Do No Harm

Nonmaleficence was the earliest ethical principle in the hierarchy of bioethics. There was a simple reason. Early physicians could do nothing to cure patients because there was no science available. Early physicians did what they believed was correct, but often there was harm to the patient. President George Washington in his final days was treated with the application of leeches. The belief was that the leeches would suck out the poisons in the blood and help a patient recover. Diseases and their causes were unknown in earlier times. It is not known if the loss of blood from President Washington's body in fact hastened his demise. Medical treatment was empirical. Although the argument could be made that the president's physician believed that he was beneficent in his treatment, the treatment provided possibly caused harm. Another nonmaleficent method of care was the laying on of hands, where a physician's touch did no further harm but provided comfort to the patient. Even in movies about the frontier, when a woman was about to deliver a baby, the physician called out to the husband to boil some water. There was no need for the boiling water because the reality was that disinfection practices were unknown at the time. The real purpose was to get the husband out of the room, occupying his time boiling water to keep him from getting in the way of the physician or midwife.

Beneficence – Do What Benefits the Patient

As physicians discovered science and disinfection, they were able to benefit patients by providing care. During the Civil War, military surgeons became adept at limb amputation without the benefit of general anesthetic to remove potentially fatal gangrenous limbs. Patients went into shock and if they recovered rather than died, the limb was surgically removed, the stump cauterized, and wounded soldiers lived another day. When physicians were able to cure problems, then beneficence rose in the hierarchy of ethical principles and along with nonmaleficence became the risks versus benefits decision-making analysis that was the obligation of the physician.

Autonomy—The Patient Makes the Choice To Consent To or To Refuse Recommended Treatment

Many ethicists regard autonomy as the top ethical principle. Beauchamp and Childress argue that in fact there is no hierarchy because biomedical decision making usually does not involve all 4 principles.[21] It is important to understand how autonomy evolved. Health care in the past and in major areas of the modern world exists in a system of paternalism. In other words, the physician made all medical decisions. The patient was left out of the dialogue except to be told that something had to be done and the procedure would be done on a certain date. Most patients responded by saying, "do whatever is necessary, you're the Doc."

Justice

Often the term, *distributive justice* or *for the common good*, is used. This element of biomedical ethics addresses the allocation of resources to a finite group of individuals. A Health Maintenance Organization (HMO) is an example of the process. If an HMO has enrolled several patients, it assumes the responsibility to provide the health care necessary for all of their patients. Insurance premiums are the funding source for operation of the HMO. The HMO needs office space, an acute care hospital with an emergency department, clinical laboratory and radiography capabilities, food services, medical staff, nursing staff, and other personnel from office workers to housekeepers. What if 1 of the thousands of enrolled patients has a disease that cannot be cured by ordinary means? Perhaps costly experimental drugs are the only chance for a cure. For an HMO to obtain the medications for this 1 patient, it must use an extraordinary amount of expense. Here are some questions to consider:

1. Will the cost have an impact on the provision of medical services to other patients?
2. Why should an HMO purchase a medication that could be labeled experimental to provide treatment to 1 individual, despite that use of the medication is not yet standard of care?
3. If the value of services provided to 1 patient decreases the level of care to all the patients, is that fair allocation of resources?

These are examples of questions to consider in trying to make a determination of what meets the best interest of this patient and all the patients of an HMO. The biomedical ethics factors of nonmaleficence, beneficence, and autonomy in the decision-making calculus should also be considered.

HAS AUTONOMY PREVAILED AS THE BASIS FOR INFORMED CONSENT IN GREAT BRITAIN?

Paternalism is still highly regarded in most areas of the world, and in Great Britain the change from paternalism to autonomy occurred when the General Medical Council ruled that the Bolam test was inapplicable to the informed consent process. Attorney J. Mitchell stated the facts of the case: "A consultant anesthetist gave a diclofenac suppository for postoperative pain to a patient having four teeth extracted under general anaesthesia in the dental surgery. He did not seek the patient's specific consent preoperatively for use of the suppository but told her afterward what he had done."[23] Unfortunately, the suppository was misplaced in the patient's vagina rather than in the rectum. "Charged before the professional conduct committee of the General Medical Council with failure to obtain informed consent and assault, the anaesthetist was found guilty of serious professional misconduct and admonished. This decision has far reaching implications and has caused great concern."[23] In addition, the dentist was also charged and found guilty of serious professional conduct, even though he had nothing to do with the suppository incident. He was "aggrieved" about the findings.[22] The Bolam test states "that a doctor is not negligent if he or she acts in accordance with a practice accepted at the time by a responsible body of medical opinion, even though other doctors may adapt a different practice."[24] In Western civilization, autonomy has come to the forefront through the doctrine of informed consent or refusal. Autonomy now gives the patient the major role in decision making in Great Britain.

NUREMBERG TRIALS – NUREMBERG, GERMANY

During World War II, Nazi physicians conducted experiments on concentration camp prisoners without their consent. Most of the participants of these experiments died or were permanently crippled. After the German surrender, the American military tribunal conducted the Nuremberg Trials beginning on December 9, 1946.[25]

In 1948, the Nuremberg Code was established based on the findings of the tribunal to address the issue of *permissible medical experiments*. There are 10 standards in the Nuremberg Code; 4 standards are listed:

1. The voluntary consent of the human subject is absolutely essential.
2. The experiment should be so conducted as to avoid all unnecessary physical and mental suffering and injury.
3. The degree of risk to be taken should never exceed that determined by human importance of the problem to be solved by the experiment.
4. During the course of the experiment the scientist in charge must be prepared to terminate the experiment at any stage, if he has probable cause to believe, in the exercise of good faith, superior skill and careful judgment required of him, that a continuation of the experiment is likely to result in injury, disability, or death to the experimental subject.[26]

TUSKEGEE STUDY (1932–1972) – TUSKEGEE, ALABAMA

The US Public Health Service conducted a study of 600 African American men. During the 40 years of the study, the men with syphilis were monitored. The test subjects were never told of their disease. The development of penicillin occurred in the twentieth century, initially discovered by Alexander Fleming in 1928. It was used by the United States and Britain to treat soldiers with syphilis as early as 1944. Unfortunately, the Tuskegee test subjects were never given the cure and most of the subjects were dead or debilitated, and the disease had been transferred to spouses and families over generations who were also denied penicillin to cure the disease until the study was halted in 1973. The study was a public embarrassment and President Bill Clinton apologized to the participants and their families for this atrocity. Again, this study lacked informed consent just as the Nazi atrocities and experiments were exposed after World War II.[27]

WILLOWBROOK STATE SCHOOL – NEW YORK

Willowbrook State School in Staten Island, New York, housed and cared for children who were mentally disabled. Dr Saul Krugman from the New York University School of Medicine and his coworkers began conducting hepatitis studies there in 1955 and continued for more than 15 years. Children with developmental disabilities were deliberately given hepatitis to see the effects of gamma-globulin therapy.[28]

JEWISH CHRONIC DISEASE HOSPITAL – NEW YORK

These studies involved the injection of foreign, live cancer cells into 22 senile patients who were hospitalized with various chronic debilitating diseases in 1963. Patients were not told that they would receive cancer cells because the researchers thought it would unnecessarily frighten them.[28]

MELANOMA TRANSFER

Beecher, in his classic article "Ethics and Clinical Research," published in *The New England Journal of Medicine* in 1966,[29] listed 3 known effective treatments deliberately withheld from the patients in research studies. He presented 22 examples of research done without full informed consent. Beecher's publication provided evidence of questionable research and led to the revealing of other evidence through the media and other researchers. He also presented the Jewish Chronic Disease Hospital research and gave the example of a transfer of a melanoma surgically from a terminally ill daughter to her mother to understand cancer immunity and antibody production. The daughter died the next day. The primary implant was widely excised on the 24th day after it had been placed. The mother died from diffuse metastatic melanoma on the 451st day after transplantation.[29] Kopp, in an article entitled, "Henry Knowles Beecher and the Development of Informed Consent in Anesthesia Research,"[30] made the following statement about Dr Beecher: "He questioned the science behind Nazi experiments conducted in concentration camps and extended the question to those conducted by other physicians and scientists. In doing so, he became convinced that a study to be scientifically valid, must be ethical from its inception."[30]

All of these misdirected experiments on human beings had the common element of lack of informed consent. The patients did not have the autonomy to consent or to refuse to the experiment. This major problem was addressed by the federal and state courts in 2 landmark decisions in the same year 1972.

THE COURTS

The federal appellate court held that a patient's true consent is an informed exercise of choice, with an opportunity to evaluate knowledgeably the options, risks, and alternatives to treatment.[31]

The California Supreme Court held that the physician had a duty to disclose all material information to make a decision, including possible alternatives; inherent known risk of death or complications that might occur must be explained in lay terms; and a reasonably prudent person in the patient's position would have decided to consent if adequately informed of all significant perils.[32]

Throughout history, persons with disabilities have been treated cruelly and the perpetrators had no real understanding of the individual's condition. Only after World War II did society notice a total disregard for a person's autonomy in medical experimentation and the horrors of war. In addition, although physicians cared for their patients by not harming them further, the development of scientific knowledge led to physicians actually being able to do some good. Years of nonmaleficence and beneficence further disadvantaged patients' drive for autonomy and whether to consent or to refuse treatment based on knowledge of material facts as opposed to the standard of paternalism, the health care philosophy that believes that decisions on health are best left in the hands of those providing care.

According to the American Psychiatric Association, the *DSM-5* was introduced in 2013 and contained the first major revision after 2 decades. Health care professionals in the United States and much of the world use the *DSM-5* as the authoritative guide for the diagnosis of mental disorders.[33]

DIAGNOSTIC AND STATISTICAL MANUAL OF MENTAL DISORDERS (FIFTH EDITION): SIGNIFICANT CHANGES

There were 2 major changes in the *DSM-5* definitions that define certain developmental disabilities.

Intellectual Disability

The term, *intellectual disability*, replaced the previous label of *mental retardation.* Mental retardation is virtually an obsolete term, replaced in state laws and in definitions used by advocacy associations. The American Association on Mental Retardation is now the American Association on Intellectual and Developmental Disabilities.[33]

Autism Spectrum Disorder

In the *Diagnostic and Statistical Manual of Mental Disorders* (Fourth Edition), autistic disorder, Asperger disorder, Rett disorder, and childhood disintegrative disorder are individually defined diagnostic categories.[34]

In *DSM-5*, the diagnoses are collectively under the category of ASDs. Asperger disorder is now referred to as *mild autism*.[33]

PREVALENCE

Prevalence is the proportion of a population who have a specific characteristic in a given time period – in medicine, typically a condition or a risk factor. The Centers for Disease Control conducted a new study of US children to determine the prevalence of developmental disabilities over a 12-year period (1997–2008). Data from National Health Interviews were gathered over a 12-year period 1997 to 2008 on children aged 3 to 17. Prevalence of developmental disabilities increased from 12.84% to 15.04%. The investigators concluded that developmental disabilities are common and were reported in approximately 1 in 6 children in the United States in 2006 to 2008. Over the 12-year period, the prevalence of developmental disabilities increased 17.1% (1.8 million more children).[35]

DEFINITIONS OF DEVELOPMENTAL DISABILITY

The Developmental Disabilities Assistance and Bill of Rights Act of 2000 (P.L. 106–402) defines a developmental disability as a severe chronic disability of an individual that

- Is attributable to a mental or physical impairment or combination of mental and physical impairments
- Is manifested before the individual attains age 22
- Is likely to continue indefinitely
- Results in substantial functional limitations in 3 or more of the following areas of major life activity: self-care, receptive and expressive language, learning, mobility, self-direction, capacity for independent living, and economic self-sufficiency
- Reflects an individual's need for a combination and sequence of special, interdisciplinary, or generic services; individualized supports; or other forms of assistance that are of lifelong or extended duration and are individually planned and coordinated

An individual from birth to age 9, who has a substantial developmental delay or specific congenital or acquired condition, may be considered to have a developmental disability without meeting 3 or more of the criteria described previously if the individual, without services and supports, has a high probability of meeting those criteria later in life.[3]

Under state law, the definition may be altered from the federal definition. In federal law, a developmental disability originates before an individual attains 22 years of age, whereas under California law, a developmental disability originates before an individual attains 18 years of age. California law also specifies that "the term shall include intellectual disability, cerebral palsy, epilepsy, and autism"[36] (**Table 2**).

CALIFORNIA WELFARE AND INSTITUTIONS CODE

In section 4512 (a), of Chapter 1.6, General Provisions, of the California Welfare and Institutions Code, "developmental disability" means a disability that originates before an individual attains 18 years of age; continues, or can be expected to continue, indefinitely; and constitutes a substantial disability for that individual. As defined by the Director of Developmental Services, in consultation with the Superintendent of Public Instruction, this term includes intellectual disability, cerebral palsy, epilepsy, and autism. This term also includes disabling conditions found closely related to intellectual disability or requiring treatment similar to that required for individuals with an intellectual disability but not including other handicapping conditions that are solely physical in nature.

INTELLECTUAL DISABILITY

Intellectual disability (ID) involves impairments of general mental abilities that impact adaptive functioning in three domains, or areas. These domains determine how well an individual copes with everyday tasks: The conceptual domain includes skills in language, reading, writing, math, reasoning, knowledge, and memory. The social domain refers to empathy, social judgment, interpersonal communication skills, the ability to make and retain friendships, and similar capacities. The practical domain centers on self-management in areas such as personal care, job responsibilities, money management, recreation, and organizing school and work tasks. While intellectual disability does not have a specific age requirement, an individual's symptoms must begin during the developmental period and are diagnosed based on the severity of deficits in adaptive functioning. The disorder is considered chronic and often co-occurs with other mental conditions like depression, attention-deficit/hyperactivity disorder, and autism spectrum disorder.[33]

Table 2
Major categories of developmental disabilities

Category*	2007 Number	Percent	2014 Number	Percent
Intellectual disability	143,965	74.4	158,639	67.6
ASD	36,952	19.1	68,832	29.3
Epilepsy	37,887	19.6	38,789	16.5
Cerebral palsy	34,646	17.9	35,691	15.2
Diagnostics categories	193,522	100	234,831	100

* Some clients may have more than 1 category of disability.
Data from California Department of Developmental Services. Fact book. 11th edition; 2008; and California Department of Developmental Services. Fact book. 12th edition; 2015.

COMPREHENSIVE ASSESSMENT

DSM-5 emphasizes the need to use both clinical assessment and standardized testing of intelligence when diagnosing intellectual disability, with the severity of impairment based on adaptive functioning rather than IQ test scores alone. By removing IQ test scores from the diagnostic criteria, but still including them in the text description of intellectual disability, DSM-5 ensures that they are not over-emphasized as the defining factor of a person's overall ability, without adequately considering functioning levels. This is especially important in forensic cases. It is important to note that IQ or similar standardized test scores should still be included in an individual's assessment. In DSM-5, intellectual disability is considered to be approximately two standard deviations or more below the population, which equals an IQ score of about 70 or below. The assessment of intelligence across three domains (conceptual, social, and practical) will ensure that clinicians base their diagnosis on the impact of the deficit in general mental abilities on functioning needed for everyday life. This is especially important in the development of a treatment plan. The updated criteria will help clinicians develop a fuller, more accurate picture of patients, a critical step in providing them with effective treatment and services.[33]

Intellectual disability can be a minor or major problem for an individual (**Table 3**).[37] The condition must manifest prior to age 18 and can start before birth and includes Down syndrome, fetal alcohol syndrome, fragile X syndrome, other genetic conditions, and birth defects. Causative issues could manifest during birth or shortly after birth. Lastly, intellectual disability can occur later from trauma, cerebral vascular changes, or even infections.[38]

AUTISM SPECTRUM DISORDER

DSM-5 provides the current terminology for ASD:

People with ASD tend to have communication deficits, such as responding inappropriately in conversations, misreading nonverbal interactions, or having difficulty building friendships appropriate to their age. In addition, people with ASD may be overly dependent on routines, highly sensitive to changes in their environment, or intensely focused on inappropriate items. Again, the symptoms of people with ASD will fall on a continuum, with some individuals showing mild symptoms and others having much more severe symptoms.[33]

The National Institute of Mental Health elaborates on ASD stating that "the term 'spectrum' refers to the wide range or symptoms, skills, and levels of impairment or

Table 3 Level of intellectual disability: January 2014		
Category	Number	Percentage of Total
No intellectual disability	76,192	32.4
Mild	82,964	35.3
Moderate	34,048	14.5
Severe	14,539	6.2
Profound	9503	4
Unspecified	17,585	7.5
Total	234,831	100

Data from California Department of Developmental Services. Fact book. 12th edition; 2015.

disability that children with ASD can have."[39,40] Although there is media and anecdotal information on the causes of autism, there is no conclusive evidence of any particular causative agent, while research looks at mutation of genes rather than a specific genetic code and the possibility of multiple environmental factors.

JUDICIAL PROCEEDINGS

In 2002, various petitioners filed claims for vaccine injuries resulting in ASD or similar neurodevelopmental disorder against the Secretary of Health and Human Services. If the petitioners prevailed, they were entitled to payment through the National Vaccine Injury Compensation Program. They believed that thimerosal (Merthiolate), a mercury compound vaccine preservative, found in some vaccines prior to 2001, caused ASD. Proceedings continued until 2011 and were called the Omnibus Autism Proceeding. The courts ruled against the petitioners and all appeals were exhausted, resulting in the Petitioners' Steering Committee disbanding. The Office of the Special Masters never found a nexus between the thousands of claims and a cause of ASD in 9 years of court proceedings.[41]

EPILEPSY

Epilepsy is the tendency to have seizures and a seizure is a transient episode of central nervous system dysfunction. "Epilepsy occurs when permanent changes in brain tissue cause the brain to be too excitable or jumpy. The brain sends out abnormal signals. This results in repeated, unpredictable seizures. (A single seizure that does not happen again is not epilepsy.)"[33]

According to an Institute of Medicine (IOM) 2012 report, *Epilepsy Across the Spectrum: Promoting Health and Understanding*, after migraine, stroke, and Alzheimer disease, epilepsy is the fourth most common neurologic disorder. Furthermore, approximately 150,000 new cased are diagnosed annually in the United States, adding to the estimated 2.2 million people with epilepsy. Surprisingly, the 2 age groups in the population to develop epilepsy are children and older adults. IOM's report states the following: "Approximately 1 in 26 people will develop epilepsy in their lives."[42]

Classification

The condition of epilepsy, not the seizure itself, is responsible for a deterioration.[42] Previously, epilepsy was thought to be a chronic, progressive condition. The historical belief was when a person had 1 seizure a second seizure would ultimately occur as the progression continued. The classification of the types of seizures includes major motor, minor motor, myoclonic, febrile, and simple and complex partial seizures (**Box 1**). There are several antiepileptic medications available by prescription with different mechanisms of action, including sodium channel, calcium channel blocker and calcium inhibitor, GABAergic, glutamate, and neuronal potassium channel openers (**Table 4**). Many of the medications still in use were developed prior to 1978. The newer medications were not approved by the Food and Drug Administration (FDA) until after 1993 (**Table 5**).

The International League Against Epilepsy (ILAE) commissioned a task force to develop a practical (operational) definition of epilepsy. The results were published and adopted as a position of the ILAE. A major change in the definition is that epilepsy is now called a disease rather than a disorder.[43] The ILAE-approved definition was published in 2014:

A person is considered to have epilepsy if they meet any of the following conditions: 1. At least 2 unprovoked (or reflex) seizures occurring greater than 24 hours

Box 1
Types of seizures

Major motor seizures – tonic-clonic (grand mal)

Minor motor seizures – absence (petit mal)

Myoclonic seizures – short episodes of spasms and contractions

Febrile seizures – during childhood up to age 6 from high fever

Simple partial seizures – abnormal electrical activity in a specific area of the brain

Complex partial seizures – abnormal electrical activity a specific area of the brain but may expand to both cerebral hemispheres

apart. 2. One unprovoked (or reflex) seizure and a probability of further seizures similar to the general recurrence risk (at least 60%) after two unprovoked seizures, occurring over the next 10 years. 3. Diagnosis of an epilepsy syndrome. Epilepsy is considered to be resolved for individuals who had an age-dependent epilepsy syndrome but are now past the applicable age or those who have remained seizure-free for the last 10 years, with no seizure medicines for the last 5 years.[43]

CEREBRAL PALSY

The National Institutes of Health defines cerebral palsy: "The term cerebral palsy refers to any one of a number of neurologic disorders that appear in infancy or early childhood and permanently affect body movement and muscle coordination but don't worsen over time. Even though cerebral palsy affects muscle movement, it isn't caused by problems in the muscles or nerves. It is caused by abnormalities in parts of the brain that control muscle movements."[44]

There are several classification methods for cerebral palsy:

1. One method is by severity usually described as mild, moderate, or severe.
2. Another classification describes which body parts are affected. This is a cerebral palsy classification based on topographic location of the affected area of the body[45] (**Table 6**).
3. Motor classification is the third way to describe cerebral palsy. Neurologic centers affected in the process leading to cerebral palsy provide a guide to describe some of the conditions, which result in anatomic limitations. When an individual has spasticity in the extremities, the condition is based upper motor neuron damage

Table 4					
Antiepileptic drugs by categories of action and medications					
Antiepileptic Medications					
Sodium Channel	**Calcium Channel Blocker**	**Calcium Inhibitor**	**GABAergic**	**Glutamate**	**Neuronal Potassium Channel Openers**
Phenytoin	Ethosuximide	Acetazolaride	Barbiturates	Febriamate	Retigabine
Carbamazepine			Benzodiazepines	Levetiracetan	
Oxcarbazepedine			Gabapentin	Peramprel	
Zonisamide			Pregabalin	Topiramate	
Lamotrigine			Tiagabine		
Eslicarbazepine			Valproate		

Table 5
Food and Drug Administration–approved antiepileptic drugs

	Major Motor	Minor Motor	Myoclonic	Febrile	Simple Partial	Complex Partial
Antiepileptic medications FDA approved prior to 1978						
Phenytoin	X	—	—	—	X	X
Phenobarbital	X	—	—	X	X	X
Carbamazepine	X	—	—	—	X	X
Ethosuximide	—	X	—	—	—	—
Valproic acid	X	X	X	—	—	—
Primidone	X	X	X	—	X	—
Clonazepam	—	X	X	—	—	—
Antiepileptic medications FDA approved after 1993						
Gabapentin	X	—	—	—	X	X
Lamotrigine	X	—	—	—	X	X
Zonisamide	—	—	—	—	X	X
Levetiracetam	—	—	—	—	X	X
Oxcarbazepine	—	—	—	—	X	X
Topiramate	—	—	—	—	X	X

involving the pyramidal tracts. The corticospinal tract conducts impulses from the brain to the spinal cord, whereas the corticobulbar tract impulses go to the brainstem and cranial nerves. The corticospinal damage often results in an extensor plantar reflex, which is retained beyond infancy (12–24 months), called the Babinski sign[46] (**Table 7**).

Often the classification of developmental disabilities is misunderstood. Intellectual disability is diagnostic in itself and is not a portion of the definition of ASD, epilepsy, or cerebral palsy. An individual may have 1 developmental disability or may have more than 1 developmental disability; however, each is a separate diagnostic category. As an example, if an individual has cerebral palsy, by definition that individual does not have an intellectual disability unless it is a concomitant developmental disability for that person. Often a patient with cerebral palsy may have difficulties speaking or being understood, but it is not a condition of intellectual disability, it is a condition of cerebral palsy. Similarly, a person may have epilepsy and any other separate developmental disability, such as intellectual disability, ASD, or cerebral palsy, but the other developmental disabilities are not a result of the epilepsy but a separate diagnostic category.

Table 6
Cerebral palsy—topographic classification (body parts affected)

Monoplegia	One extremity
Paraplegia	Two lower extremities
Hemiplegia	Two extremities – one side of body
Quadriplegia	All 4 extremities

Table 7		
Types of cerebral palsy—motor classification		
Spastic—pyramidal	Hypertonic muscle function 70%–80% of cerebral palsy cases Pyramidal tract – upper motor neuron damage	
Nonspastic— extrapyramidal	Hypotonic muscle function 20% of cerebral palsy cases Extrapyramidal – neuron damage outside of the pyramidal tracts	

SUMMARY

A review of the ADA of 1990 and its amendments, the latest in 2008, is useful to understand because they have implications in the practice of dentistry. Since 1992, dental offices are considered places of public accommodation; therefore, all the ramifications under federal regulations apply to dental offices as far as seeing patients with disabilities and making offices and buildings compliant to accommodate patients.

The word, disability, has several connotations. This article, in part, reviews the factors in the determination of a disability as well as the definitions of developmental disabilities. Recently, *DSM-5* and the American Association on Intellectual and Developmental Disabilities have replaced the outdated term, mental retardation, with the term, intellectual disability. Another *DSM-5* change is the term, ASD, for a wide variety of autistic diagnoses replacing autism and changing the term Asperger disorder to mild autism.

The term, disability, means different things to different people. Dentists may first think of some patients who have developmental and other disabilities. As practice owners, they think of all the access issues government has put in place make operating a dental office seem overregulated. The stand-alone term, disability, is a conundrum and carries with it many meanings. This article focuses on the ADA and a discussion of several diagnostic categories of developmental disabilities to increase understanding of these topics and the public dentists serve and, hopefully, Adrian Killoran can still go to school with his friends and continue to achieve.

REFERENCES

1. Hamptons, New York School wants to block student with down syndrome on 1st Day by genevieve shaw brown, ABC News. Available at: http://abcnews.go.com/Lifestyle/hamptons-york-school-block-student-syndrome-1st-day/print?id=33431544.
2. U.S. Department of Health and Human Services. Oral health in America: a report of the surgeon general. U.S. Department of Health and Human Services, National Institute of Dental and Craniofacial Research, National Institutes of Health; 2000.
3. AwDA enacted into law on July 26, 1990, P.L. 101-336; 42 U.S.C. 12102. AwDA Title III Regulations, 28 CFR Part 36; AwDA Amendments Act of 2008 (Pub. L. No. 110-325).
4. American Dental Association Division of Legal Affairs. Americans with disabilities act: questions & answers. American Dental Association; 1992.
5. U.S. Department of Justice. A guide to disability rights laws, 2009. Available at: www.ada.gov/cguide.pdf.
6. Fact Sheet on the EEOC's Final Regulations Implementing the ADAAA. U.S. Equal Employment Opportunity Commission. 2011. Available at: http://www.eeoc.gov/laws/regulations/adaaa_fact_sheet.cfm.

7. Benfer EA. The ADA Amendments Act: an overview of recent changes to the Americans with disabilities act. Am Constitution Soc for Law and Policy; 2009. p. 1–18.
8. U.S. Department of Justice. The ADA and City Governments: Common Problems. Civil Rights Division, Disability Rights Section. Available at: http://www.ada.gov/comprob.pdf.
9. 28 C.F.R. §§35.130(b)(7).
10. Bragdon v. Abbott 524 U.S. 624 (1998).
11. Olmstead v. L.C. 527 U.S. 581 (1999).
12. 42 U.S. Code § 12181.
13. 28 CFR Part 36. Under §36.101.
14. 42 U.S.C. 12181.
15. A Settlement Agreement between the United States of America Department of Justice and the University of Medicine and Dentistry of New Jersey. Available at: http://www.ada.gov/undnj_sa.htm.
16. Parr v. LL Drive Inn Restaurant 96 F. Supp.2d 1065 (D. Haw. 2000).
17. Franklin KA, Thompson MO. Reducing the risk of an AwDA lawsuit. J Calif Dent Assoc 2013;41(9):689–93.
18. Definition of Intellectual Disability, American Association on Intellectual and Developmental Disabilities (AAIDD) http://www.aaidd.org/content_100.cfm?navID=21.
19. Perspectives on the historical treatment of people with disabilities. Teaching for diversity and social justice. 2nd edition. Routledge; 2007. Appendix 14C.
20. Blumberg JA. Brief history of the salem witch trials. Smithsonian Mag 2007;1–3.
21. Beauchamp T, Childress J. Principles of biomedical ethics. 7th edition. New York: Oxford University Press; 2013.
22. Lawrence DJ. The four principles of biomedical ethics: a foundation for current bioethical debate. J Chiropr Humanit 2007;14:34–40.
23. Mitchell J. A fundamental problem of consent. BMJ 1995;310:43–6.
24. Bolam v. Friern Hospital Management Committee 1957;1WLR 582.
25. History of ethics. Available at: http://www.cgu.edu/pages/1722.asp.
26. The nuremberg code. BMJ 1996;7070(313):1448.
27. Brand AM. Racism and research: the case of the Tuskegee Institute syphilis study. Hastings Center Magazine 1978;1–3.
28. Dunn CM, Chadwick G. Protecting study volunteers in research: a manual for investigative sites. Center Watch, Inc., University of Rochester Medical Center; 1999. p. 2–4.
29. Beecher HK. Ethics and clinical research. N Engl J Med 1966;274(24):1354–60.
30. Kopp VJ. Henry Knowles Beecher and the development of informed consent in anesthesia research. Anesthesiology 1999;90(6):1756–65.
31. Canterbury v. Spence 464 F2d 772 (DCCir 1972).
32. Cobbs v. Grant 8 C3d 229 (1972).
33. American Psychiatric Association. Diagnostic and statistical manual of mental disorders. 5th edition. Washington, DC: American Psychiatric Association; 2013.
34. Available at: http://www.autism-society.org/.
35. Centers for Disease Control. Trends in the prevalence of developmental disabilities in US children. CDC Report 1997–2008.
36. Developmental Disability. California Welfare and Institutions Code §4512.
37. Surabian SR. Developmental disabilities and understanding the needs of patients with mental retardation and Down syndrome. J Calif Dent Assoc 2001;29(6):415–23.

38. Definition of Intellectual Disability, American Association on Intellectual and Developmental Disabilities (AAIDD). Available at: http://www.aaidd.org/content_100.cfm?navID=21.
39. Surabian SR. Dentistry's intrinsic link to provision of services for persons with disabilities. J Calif Dent Assoc 2013;41(9):677–88.
40. Available at: http://www.nimh.nih.gov/health/topics/autism-spectrum-disorders-asd/index.shtml.
41. Available at: http://www.uscfc.uscourts.gov/sites/default/files/autism/Autism%20Update%201%2012%.
42. Fisher RS, Acevedo C, Arzimanoglou A, et al. A practical clinical definition of epilepsy. Epilepsia 2014;55(4):475–82.
43. Available at: http://www.epilepsy.com/article/2014/4/revised-definition-epilepsy.
44. Available at: http://www.ninds.nih.gov/disorders/cerebral_palsy/cerebral_palsy.htm
45. Surabian SR. Developmental disabilities: epilepsy, cerebral palsy and autism. J Calif Dent Assoc 2001;29(6):424–32.
46. Guyton JE, Hall JE. Textbook of medical physiology. 13th edition. Philadelphia: W.B. Saunders; 2015.

Making Treatment of Special Needs Patients an Important Part of Your Growing Dental Practice

Craig C. Spangler, DDS, FSCDA[a,b,*]

KEYWORDS

- Special needs patients • Private practice • Hospital dentistry
- General practice residency • Continuum of care

KEY POINTS

- Many dentists who have completed hospital-based, general practice residency programs do not use all of the skills they have learned in their subsequent private practice careers.
- There is a tremendous need for dental treatment of patients with special needs in every community, especially with the aging population and increased longevity.
- Hospital affiliation can provide an opportunity to provide quality care for special needs patients, while creating visibility and enhancing the professional reputation of the dentist.
- Working with dental specialists in treating patients with special needs not only provides excellent treatment but also provides an opportunity to foster professional partnerships and practice growth.
- There is a place in a community for a dentist who wants ongoing relationships with special needs patients, to provide excellent treatment, and be paid as they would for any other patient.

Today many young dentists are looking to make their practices satisfying in ways other than only the financial rewards of dentistry. Some of these new practitioners have gained additional training in diagnosis and treatment of medically and physically challenging patients. Quite often, those dentists with additional training have found the treatment of special needs patients to be a gratifying application of the skills they learned in their postgraduate training. There is an opportunity to grow a practice through seeking those patients who require this type of care and develop the long-term relationships that are beneficial to both doctor and patients. As our society ages, and patients live longer, there will be demand for the dentist who has the

Disclosure Statement: The author has nothing to disclose.
[a] St Joseph Mercy Oakland, 44405 Woodward Ave, Pontiac, MI 48341, USA; [b] Private Practice of General Dentistry, 4050 W. Maple Rd, Suite 220, Bloomfield Hills, MI 48301, USA
* 4050 West Maple Road, Suite 220, Bloomfield Hills, MI 48301.
E-mail address: cspang@comcast.net

http://dx.doi.org/10.1016/j.cden.2016.02.009
dental.theclinics.com

training, desire, and ability to work with these special needs patients. This level of special care will be demonstrated to family and caregivers, and soon they will want to be patients in that kind of practice also. Word of mouth, along with the visibility that comes from treating patients with special needs, creates an opportunity to create trusting relationships with potential patients. By taking care of those who are most vulnerable, a dentist will earn a reputation as a caring, dedicated dentist who is interested in doing what is best for his or her patients.

THERE ARE DENTISTS TRAINED TO DO THIS

Today we have many general dentists who have completed hospital-based general dental residency programs.[1] These programs have been in existence for more than 50 years and are offered throughout the United States. This optional year of training is designed to give residents clinical and didactic opportunities that go beyond their training in dental school. Many recent graduates lack significant clinical experiences in comparison with graduates of previous years. Even more significantly, dental schools today are unable to provide the comprehensive treatment experiences for dental students in treating people with medically or physically compromising conditions. Although there may be some exposure to special needs patients, treatment planning and the clinical treatment of these challenging patients is an experience that most students will not receive in school. As dental schools provide fewer clinical experiences, the optional year of training is even more important in the development of the new dentist. Some states, such as New York, have recognized that additional training in all areas of dentistry is now essential to a recent graduate.[2]

In many programs accredited by the Commission on Dental Accreditation (CODA), treatment of patients with special needs is an important part of their curriculum. These patients include medically compromised, physically compromised, and geriatric patients. The goal of a hospital based general practice residency, as defined by CODA's goals, is to train general dentists who are knowledgeable in treating patients with special needs.[3] This year or two of training comes at a time when young dentists are defining who they will be as dentists and as people. Yet this specially trained group of general dentists usually goes into private practice and blends in with all the other practitioners. They do not take advantage of many of the skills that they were taught or the experiences that they had in the general dental residency program. Quite often they do not recognize the depth and breadth of their training and how it is has given them additional expertise in comparison with their peers.

Under pressure from senior dentists, practice consultants, and crushing student loan debt, they all too readily accept a model for a successful private practice and attempt to emulate that model. It may be the cosmetic practice or the sleep medicine practice or some other concept. The focus of this niche practice will change and will come and go with time. Although certainly there is an opportunity to build a practice only based on treating patients with special needs, there is another way that is more practical for young dentists. They can make the treatment of patients with special needs an inclusive and integral part of their practice, as all areas of our country are in need of dentists to treat those with special needs.

THERE IS DEMAND FOR SPECIAL NEEDS DENTISTRY

In the early 1980s, many states closed institutions where mentally and physically impaired patients were in residence. When a child was born with special needs, parents were advised to give up physical custody of the child. The child would then be institutionalized with the rationale that they could be best taken care of in that setting. It was thought that because of their condition, they would not be able to exist in the outside world. However, some of the institutions were found to be inadequate in many ways, to the point of neglect. This inadequacy resulted in the closing of the institutions and the deinstitutionalization of the residents.[4] The residents were placed in homes, in a community setting, that were referred to as *group homes* or *foster homes*. This placement allowed for the residents to attend special schools, sheltered workshops, and participate in other community settings that were totally new to them.

This placement also meant that many of the medical, dental, and allied health services that were necessary, and important, needed to be found in the community. At the 1984 American Academy of Dentistry for the Handicapped meeting in Atlanta, Dr Arthur Nowak[5], the author of *Dentistry for the Handicapped Patient* (C.V. Mosby Co, 1976), showed his concerns about the future success of deinstitutionalization.[6] He was not convinced that the same level of medical and dental services would be available in the community as was found in the institutions. He asserted that health care providers in the institutions had expertise that could not be easily replaced. However, some residential facilities did not provide the quality medical and dental services that met the needs of these patients. In some cases, states restricted the available financial resources that limited the quality of care available to the residents and resulted in substandard treatment.

As Dr Novak suggested in his remarks, dentists in the community were not prepared to treat the needs of these patients. This lack of training resulted in many parents and caregivers going from dentist to dentist, unable to find anyone who could provide care for their patient with special needs. Often the outcome was frustration, anger, and resentment toward dentistry in general, as no one was capable of helping these challenging patients. Along with this frustration, there was a lack of any treatment philosophies or goals for the dentition of these patients. Were the goals for treatment the same as all other patients? How important was keeping their teeth for their lifetime, more important or less important because they were considered less whole than someone else? Who was going to pay for the necessary treatment?

Caregivers were justifiably concerned when a dentist might suggest that maintaining teeth was less important in these patients than any other patient. Some of this attitude was reinforced by physicians who also lacked the ability to foresee the changes that would be happening in the attitudes of the public and how rewarding community living could be for those who were deinstitutionalized.

HOW DOES A PRACTICE OFFER CARE FOR SPECIAL NEEDS PATIENTS?

Many parents and caregivers become frustrated by the lack of availability of dentists to treat patients with special needs. They frequently have made numerous phone calls, searched the Internet, and had not succeeded in finding a dentist. Sometimes the dentists, who are willing to treat special needs patients, cannot provide the services necessary for their patients. Even if they are willing, they may lack the ability, experience, or equipment to provide care for every patient. A recent study in a suburban Detroit area revealed that 80% of special needs patients 14 to 26 years of age are unable to find a dentist to treat them.[7] Situations like these lead to tremendous frustration on many levels for those seeking any type of dental care.

This situation is exactly the reason that there is an opportunity for dentists trained in treating patients with special needs to develop this skill as part of their practice. Ideally, if dentists can offer enough different modes of service delivery, they can tell a caregiver that one way or the other, we will provide care. This statement is rarely heard by a caregiver in the special needs community. However, it is realistic and achievable for dentists who have training and skills in this area.

In 1985, a concept was articulated that probably has been shown in several different forms previously.[8] Called the Continuum of Care, it is a diagrammatic representation of all the modes of dental care delivery from simplest to the most complex (**Fig. 1**). The concept is that all patients, especially those with special needs, will fit somewhere on the continuum and that everyone can be treated. Patients may be at different places on the continuum, depending on the procedure, their medical status, and their behavior. Not all dentists may be able or choose to offer all of the modalities shown, but it can be a starting point for determining how care can be delivered. This concept will create a framework for application of dentists' philosophy of care, which is discussed later in this article. For example, if the dentist thinks that radiographs are a necessity for patients at certain intervals, how will they be obtained? Patients may be cooperative for examination and scaling but not for radiographs. Perhaps this

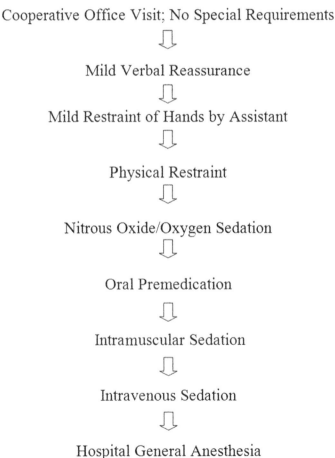

Cooperative Office Visit; No Special Requirements

⇩

Mild Verbal Reassurance

⇩

Mild Restraint of Hands by Assistant

⇩

Physical Restraint

⇩

Nitrous Oxide/Oxygen Sedation

⇩

Oral Premedication

⇩

Intramuscular Sedation

⇩

Intravenous Sedation

⇩

Hospital General Anesthesia

Fig. 1. The Continuum of care is a framework for providing dental care for patients, no matter what their special physical or mental needs so that quality of care can be delivered in the least risky environment. Each practitioner may have their own modes of treatment delivery that will fall somewhere on the continuum.

can be done with someone, with appropriate shielding, staying in the room to stabilize these patients. Or it may require a form of sedation to achieve a quality image. How important are good radiographs in treating patients? They are very important in giving these patients the same quality of services that any other patient deserves. Although it may not be easy, the answer to this question reflects the dentists' philosophy of care.

The Continuum of Care provides a starting point for dentists to plan for necessary treatment but to also reevaluate their approach to patients. Quite often patients who have major dental problems can be seen in the most intensive mode, general anesthesia in the hospital, and treated comprehensively. Once their needs are met, this is a new opportunity for the dentist to begin again. Soreness is gone; inflammation has been reduced; patients have no underlying problems (**Figs. 2** and **3**). Home care instruction and a renewed emphasis on dietary controls can improve the ongoing oral health of patients. In some cases, these patients can sometimes be seen at the other end of the continuum, with a regular office visit, and do quite well. Although dentists may not be able to provide comprehensive care in this setting, is it possible that some preventive and diagnostic care can be delivered? This care allows for an ongoing relationship with patients and caregivers and a monitoring of the medical, dental, and behavioral health of patients. It is not uncommon to have patients who are often treated with intravenous conscious sedation or general anesthesia do quite well for preventive care. Quality, definitive treatment provided in the hospital operating room can alleviate pain and problems to a point where preventive services can be simple and comfortable for patients. The concept of the Continuum of Care provides a framework for the ongoing relationship of the dentist and patients.

DEVELOPING YOUR OWN PHILOSOPHY OF CARE

Treatment of patients with special needs has all too frequently been only on an as needed basis. When a problem occurs, or someone thinks there is a problem, they are brought in for treatment. This situation has evolved because of many factors, such as payment or insurance limitations, difficulty in providing treatment, or even

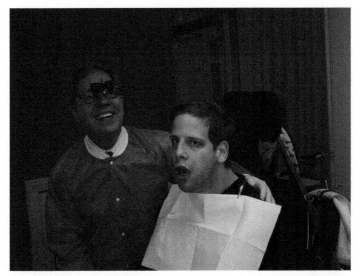

Fig. 2. A 34-year-old patient with cerebral palsy who is almost only seen in the operating room for examination, scaling, and radiographs. He is shown with the author in the dental office.

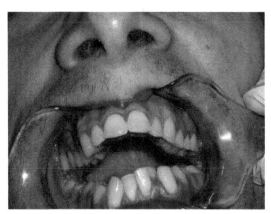

Fig. 3. The same patient's oral cavity photographed in the office about 8 weeks following his treatment under general anesthesia. Note the lack of gingival inflammation in his mouth.

finding a practitioner who wants to treat them on a regular basis. However, none of these factors takes into account what the preventive needs of patients are or what is best for them on an ongoing basis. Home care is frequently difficult to provide, and this places patients even more at risk for dental and periodontal disease. As many of these patients are on medication, or multiple medications, xerostomia can further increase the risks of dental problems. Because of these risk factors, patients with special needs are in need of more frequent examination and preventive care than other patients. Yet many times their dental needs are treated as a low priority. At best, they may schedule appointments every 6 months, similar to patients with no significant dental concerns.

Just as with any other patient, the dentist needs to be the advocate for the highest-quality treatment and ongoing care for special needs patients. There is no one else who understands the dental needs of this group of patients any more fully than experienced dentists who are well trained in treating patients with special needs. This idea is not a deviation from what should be the dentists' overall philosophy of practice but totally congruent with what they want for every patient. For example, many patients have dental benefit plans that limit frequency or payment of services in a given year. Yet, if patients require more treatment than the plan benefits, they explain the importance of treatment and make arrangements for the treatment to be done. Every patient has his or her own unique set of needs; dentists are obligated to diagnose, inform, and recommend the appropriate treatment of that patient. Why should it be any different for patients with special needs (**Fig. 4**)?

Dentists who approach their patients this way will not only be providing what is best for their patients but also creating a reputation for quality care in their community. By seeing these patients for the care they require, dentists will be busier and also more satisfied with what they are doing. Parents and caregivers will see the benefits in providing the necessary care, not being governed by limitations that do not have the patients' best interest in mind.

THIS CAN WORK IN PRIVATE PRACTICE

Too often a dentist who would treat patients with special needs makes the assumption that you must accept all forms of insurance, including the different forms of dental Medicaid. In many states, the reimbursement levels are low and the only services

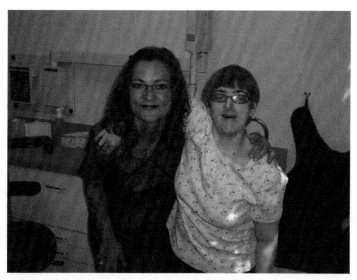

Fig. 4. A patient with Rubenstein-Taybi syndrome who has been seen in the office with oral sedation and with general anesthesia in the hospital at different times in her life depending on her cooperation and the services required. She has had a variety of dental services in the general dental office, including endodontics and fixed partial denture.

covered are extractions and other emergency procedures. After all, we would like to be able to treat all of the patients who we know require services. Yet programs that are financed by third parties, whether government or dental benefit plans, have ignored and neglected patients with special needs. Politicians who control state budgets are generally not aware of the needs of the special patient population let alone their dental needs. Should our special needs patients be penalized because of any politician or a political group's ideological budget agenda? Is not the state responsible for the welfare of these patients?

One of the basic concepts of treating patients with special needs in a general dental practice is that they pay the same as everyone else. Our interest is including them in our practice just like any other patient. When routine services are provided, they are billed at the same rate as anyone else. In the case of older adults, they may have been your patients for many years. It should be fundamental to your philosophy of practice that you will help, adapt, and support these patients as they face the challenges of aging. Yet when those services require additional time or expertise, the practitioner should charge accordingly. This idea is not any different from a difficult full-mouth rehabilitation case. It is not only 28 crowns billed as individual entities but also the complexity that goes along with rebuilding occlusion, shape, and function of the entire arch. Just as is the case the with the full-mouth rehabilitation case, there is always increased risk involved in treating people with special needs. This risk may be medical due to the complex medical status of patients. There can also be additional risk to the staff, caregivers, and the facility that can occur when resistant behavior is an issue. In order to mitigate these risks, additional fees may be necessary. This idea would also hold true for oral sedation, conscious sedation, and general anesthesia, no matter what the setting.

When caregivers are informed that you do not take Medicaid, they can take responsibility for finding out how to pay for this important service. As part of this responsibility, they will find themselves putting increased value on the service. Along with that will come better compliance with appointments, home care, and decision making that result in better care for patients. All too often, patients can suffer from caregivers who are not attentive, not well trained, and poorly paid. This situation presents an opportunity for us to help elevate the discussion of necessary services for special needs patients beyond the minimal level of services that many states provide benefits for.

Many patients do have other sources of funds available for their use. For a large number of patients who will not be able to care for themselves in the future, attorneys and accountants have helped families establish trusts for necessary future needs. Dentistry is one of the most important future needs for these patients. These funds were designated by the family to provide quality of life that they had when the family was directly taking care of these patients. Being free of pain and having a comfortable mouth that can be maintained for the future is exactly they type of benefit that these funds were designed to provide for these patients. Dentists should routinely ask if there are funds available to provide quality services that their families desire in their future plans.

Quite often dentists have treated patients with special needs for little or no fees, acknowledging that this is a charitable service. This practice is wonderful for those practitioners who choose to do this, and they are to be commended. However, if we wish to provide ongoing, quality care that is sustainable, the dentist trained in treating special needs patients must be paid a reasonable fee for treatment. By including these patients as part of a broader fee-for-service practice, there are other sources of income. Dentists do not become overly reliant on the fees generated from these patients, which allows dentists to spend the necessary time working with special needs patients, while being paid at the same rate as treating any other patient.

THE VALUE OF HOSPITAL AFFILIATION AND PRACTICE

In growing a private practice, hospital-based residency training can be an important pathway to becoming a vital member of your community. When general dentists applies for staff privileges at a hospital in or near their community, there are tremendous practice-building opportunities. Not only could you develop a way to treat patients in the operating room under general anesthesia but also to interface with the medical staff on inpatient and outpatient consultations. Dental equipment for use in the hospital today is convenient, easy to use, and relatively affordable. Whether it is a portable, handheld x-ray source or a portable dental cart, it is far easier to provide care in the hospital setting than ever before.

Every graduate of a CODA-accredited general practice residency program is familiar with how to join a hospital medical and dental staff.[9] This connection allows you to network with other health care professionals in their setting. You will become one of them, and all of the physicians have patients with dental issues. They will be looking for your guidance as to how to treat them and potentially to you as the professional to solve these patients' problems. This work will increase your profile in the community and identify you as someone who has skills that the other dentists do not have. You will become a colleague of the physicians in your community, giving you standing that almost no other general dentist has.

Even more importantly, you will meet and work with many talented nurses, administrators, and allied health professionals in the hospital. As they get to know you, they will be interested in you and your practice. They are a group that knows the value of good health, have steady income and benefits, and are frequently seeking dental information. They can become your next patient, and the hospital is a tremendous marketing opportunity for your practice. If you are visible in the hospital, you can meet many people who often are seeking a dentist. As you take the time to develop the relationships with the hospital staff, you will find that your practice will grow; these patients will become a valued source of new patient referrals. The benefits of hospital affiliation and activity are numerous and, to the growing dental practice, invaluable in increasing your professional identity in the community.

THE GROWING GERIATRIC SPECIAL NEEDS GROUP

One of the fastest growing groups of patients in any community will be the geriatric population. As baby boomers age, there will be more patients who will have tremendous dental needs. Living longer than previous generations, there will be a demand for more dental services for this group. In previous generations, older adults were mostly missing their teeth by this point, whereas today's baby boomers have expected that they will keep a full dentition throughout their lifetime. This expectation will push them to seek fixed prosthetics, such as implant-supported restorations or implant-supported prosthetics. Many of these patients will be regular patients in a practice or may be referred to the general practitioner who treats special needs patients. There will be multiple medications to manage and significant disease states that will require the knowledge that a dentist can develop during a hospital-based residency program.

Some disease states, such as dementia or other neurologic diseases, may require the same skills as those used with other special needs patients. There may be issues with behavior and cooperation that will necessitate changing treatment and how it is delivered. The expectations of family and caregivers may be very high. They still view these patients as the loved one they have always known and want what is best for them. Yet the behavior of these patients or the impact of their disease may preclude them from receiving treatment. All of the factors that create challenges for all older adults will impact these patients even more. Poor oral hygiene, lack of diet control, and additional stresses on existing teeth and restorations will provide a more challenging situation. As these patients live longer, there will be more dental challenges ahead.

Being able to serve this group creates tremendous opportunity for the growing dental practice. It will attract a new and engaged group of family and caregivers to your practice. They will get to know you and watch you treat their loved one in a quality and caring manner. Your respect for their concerns and desires will show them that you are someone unique in the dental community.

Today there is an aging population of adults mentally and physically impaired with special needs. This situation is a new development due to the medical advancements that have made daily living possible for patients with complex medical situations. In the past, medical problems would have proven fatal in early adulthood. Today, many people with special needs are living well into their 60s and 70s. This longevity presents many unique challenges for dentistry. It is easy to extract all of the teeth and rationalize the reasons for it. It is much harder to try to save the teeth that are present. Although they may not be ideal, such as have opposing teeth present, the loss of teeth can be as traumatic to someone with special needs as it is for anyone. If this person is still taking food by mouth, it is important that no one should make a rash judgment in regard to the importance of the dentition. If patients are functioning well with their dentition, the substitutes that we have available may be poor in comparison. Unless the dentist is prepared for offering a substitute, priority should be given to maintaining the current dentition.

LIMITATIONS OF MOBILE DENTISTRY

Mobile dentistry is gaining favor as a way to deliver care to patients who have physical barriers to access to dental care. This mobility is certainly a way to screen or examine many patients in a short period of time. However, there are limitations to what can be done in these scenarios. The portable equipment that can be handled by one or 2 people is lightweight and easily moved. However, this also makes it less sturdy and not substantial enough for many patients who are large. Portable vans and vehicles like motorhomes that have been converted for dentistry may have physical barriers, such as steps, that may make this option impossible for many patients. The converted motorhome also requires a substantial investment of capital, most of which is related to the ability to drive the vehicle, not the delivery of dental care.

The same technology that makes portable dentistry possible has yielded equipment that can be used in a hospital or outpatient clinic setting that is affordable and reliable. A handheld x-ray unit can be used in an office setting with a hard digital sensor. This unit can be used just as easily in the hospital or other outpatient setting. Units that run on nitrogen and generate their own Venturi-based suction can be used in any setting where piped-in nitrogen or tank nitrogen is available. These items allow the quality of care to come close to that of the dedicated dental office, yet are affordable for the hospital or dentist, especially when some of the same equipment can also be used in the office (**Figs. 5** and **6**).

However, the factor that makes this a limited mode of delivering treatment is safety. If patients are unable to come to a dental office, there are frequently several significant health factors that are limiting their mobility. This limitation may be due to age, disease, reliance on mechanical life support systems, or other severely debilitating health conditions. Most of these patients would be grouped in the American Society of Anesthesiologists' physical status 3 or 4 in regard to providing any kind of care.[10] Any physician or dentist would consider these patients higher risk. Knowing that in many long-term care facilities there is poor or limited medical care, the quality of

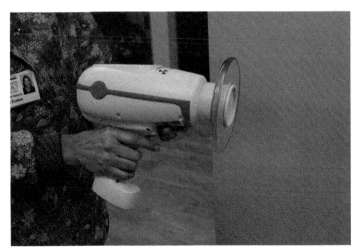

Fig. 5. A portable, handheld x-ray head that can be used with a hard sensor in settings where radiographs may not be traditionally available, such as the operating room or other areas of the hospital.

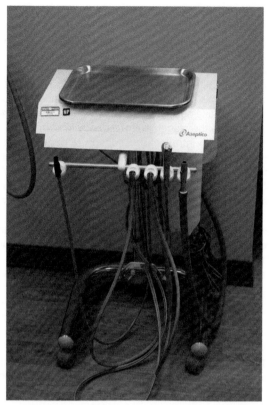

Fig. 6. A portable cart that runs off nitrogen and is a completely self-contained dental unit with suction, allowing it to be used anywhere in the hospital. (*Courtesy of* Aseptico, Inc, Woodinville, WA, with permission.)

the medical care may also be suspect. Delivering dental care to patients where medical diagnosis and treatment may be limited or incomplete puts the dentist at risk for a medical emergency during treatment.

This situation begs the question of safety in delivering treatment in a setting where there is limited support. In a dental office, a staff will have all the resources to respond to a medical emergency. Is an extraction performed at bedside truly an innocuous procedure when performed on a high-risk patient with medical care limited by state Medicaid plans or limited knowledge of the patient? It is not.

WORKING WITH DENTAL SPECIALISTS HELPS EVERYONE

In any private general dental practice, you should work with specialists for procedures that are beyond your scope of practice. You will develop a network of periodontists, oral surgeons, pediatric dentists, endodontists, and orthodontists that you think will provide the necessary, quality care for your patients. When specialists work with you in providing care, there are numerous opportunities for a mutually beneficial relationship for everyone. Quite often the general dentist learns more about how the specialist approaches a case, in comparison with how they may approach a case. The specialist may have a better treatment plan, and quite often this will provide a superior result. In addition, there may be more treatment opportunities for the general dentist, resulting in additional income. Patients, as a result of the team approach, gets a well-thought-out and synergistic plan of treatment that truly is the most beneficial solution for them.

How does this apply to special needs patients? When a patient is seen in a general dental office who has difficult or significant procedures to be undertaken, it makes sense to think about what can be done at the specialty office. For example, a patient who is missing teeth may have several options for replacement of those teeth. Could one of those options involve the placement of a dental implant? This procedure is one that would be performed with intravenous sedation or general anesthesia in an oral surgeon or periodontists office. The knowledgeable dentist's relationship with specialists makes it possible for this to be done in a safe environment while providing an excellent result. The restoration of the implant requires no local anesthesia and can frequently be done in the general dental office, even with a moderately cooperative patient.

Not all treatment will be as complex as an implant. If there is another procedure, such as a small restoration that could be done with sedation, it is logical to consider combining it with the sedation required for the implant. The oral surgeon or periodontist will be happy to give you the 10 to 15 minutes necessary for the procedure. Most importantly, they value having you in their office to become familiar with them and their staff. They are seeking referrals of your other patients who will provide them with their bread and butter: third molar extractions, periodontal surgery patients, and implant placements. Assisting their referring dentists is the most effective marketing that they can do, and your familiarity with their office can provide them with tremendous good will toward a successful referral relationship. This relationship can provide general dentists who do not perform sedation in their office with an option for treatment that can be beneficial to many special needs patients (**Figs. 7–9**).

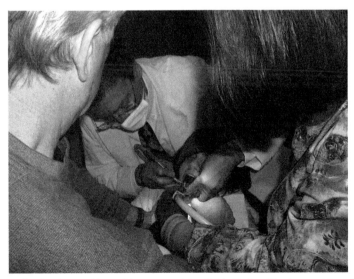

Fig. 7. An orthodontist working with a general dentist in their office to provide orthodontic treatment of a patient with Rett syndrome to align her occlusion correctly and reduce flaring of her maxillary anterior teeth due to biting her hands.

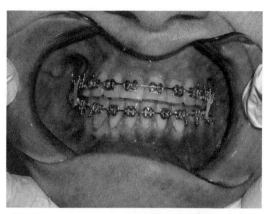

Fig. 8. The patient with Rett syndrome in orthodontic appliances during treatment. Gingival health could be maintained by good home care and frequent prophylaxis.

IMPORTANT OPPORTUNITIES FOR SPECIAL NEEDS DENTISTS

If a dentist wants to consider clinical research, a private practice that sees patients with special needs is a good place to do it. As patients may be private payers, they have the freedom to choose who will provide treatment. This option has led to long-term relationships that can provide a longitudinal perspective on what works for patients with special needs and what does not. This long-term relationship has many advantages to the patients as well. They become familiar with the routine of the office, which eases anxiety and allows for a more productive appointment. The connection can be so deep; patients with special needs will even point out an office as they drive by on their way elsewhere. The long-term relationship gives us the opportunity to evaluate what we have done and how treatment has worked out over time. There is a general lack of longitudinal studies that show how treatment of patients with special needs has been successful or unsuccessful. A private practice, where some patients have been seen for more than 20 years, can be an opportunity to show what works when ideal treatment can be delivered.

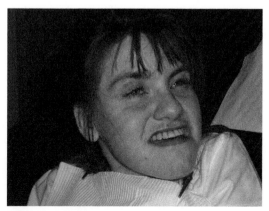

Fig. 9. A patient with Rett syndrome after treatment of the flaring of the maxillary incisors due to a finger biting habit.

SUMMARY

More than ever before there is a need for patients with special needs to have a dental home. As this population will continue to grow through medical advancements, improved health care, and longer lifespans, there will be a need for more specialized dental treatment. Dentists who have been in a general practice residency program have had the experience of working with patients who are medically and physically compromised. By including and even reaching out to them in a private practice setting, dentists can grow their practice by developing this unique service they provide. Hospital affiliation and utilization of the hospital facilities can create a desirable profile for dentists, setting them apart from the rest of the dental community. This visibility will promote the overall practice of these dentists and provide opportunities to attract new patients of all types from the community. These dentists will be seen as dentists who are caring, patient, and go out of their way to help all patients, making their practice a desirable place for everyone.

REFERENCES

1. Survey of advanced dental education 2010-11. Chicago (IL): Commission on Dental Accreditation, American Dental Association; 2012.
2. Residency Program for Dental Licensure in New York State. News and Current Issues. State of New York, Albany NY: Office of the Professions; 2009. Available at: http://www.op.nysed.gov/prof/dent/dentexampart3.htm.
3. Accreditation Standards for Advanced Education Programs in General Practice Residency. Goals. Commission on Dental Accreditation; 2010. p. 8.
4. Child Abuse at Plymouth Center. Detroit Free Press; 1977. p. 3.
5. Nowak AJ. Dentistry for the Handicapped Patient. St. Louis (MO): C.V. Mosby Co; 1976.
6. American Academy of Dentistry for the Handicapped Annual Meeting. Atlanta (GA), October 20, 1984.
7. Williams JJ, Spangler CC, Yusaf NK. Barriers to dental care for patients with special needs in an affluent metropolitan community. Special Care in Dentistry 2015; 35(4):190–6.
8. Spangler CC. Dentistry for special needs patients. Michigan Dental Association Annual Meeting. Detroit, MI, April 27, 1985
9. Accreditation Standards For Advanced Education Programs in General Practice Residency. Commission on Dental Accreditation, August 7, 2015. Available at: http://www.ada.org/~/media/CODA/Files/gpr.pdf?la=en.
10. ASA Physical classification system 2014 guidelines. Relative value guide 2016. Schaumburg, IL: American Society of Anesthesiologists; 2014.

Treatment of Orally Handicapped Edentulous Older Adults Using Dental Implants

 CrossMark

Charles Zahedi, DDS, PhD

KEYWORDS

- Edentulism • Tooth loss • Dental implants • Mini–dental implants • Osseointegration
- Prosthodontics • Overdentures

KEY POINTS

- The oral handicap of complete edentulism is the terminal outcome of a multifactorial process involving biological factors and patient-related factors. It will continue to represent a very large global health care burden for the foreseeable future.
- The fully edentulous orally handicapped older adult population has been neglected because removable acrylic dentures have been the classic therapy for complete edentulism. These soft tissue–supported prostheses do not treat alveolar bone loss or prevent disuse atrophy or pressure-mediated resorption, which are all germane to edentulism. Therefore, they are only rehabilitative, not therapeutic.
- Not replacing missing teeth with stable dentures could prevent adequate food intake.
- To address the oral handicap of complete edentulism, osseointegrated endosseous implants could be used as a therapeutic adjunct and could reduce the problem of long-term bone resorption to less than 0.1 mm per year.
- Implant-borne prostheses substantially improve the overall health and quality of life of orally handicapped fully edentulous older adults.

INTRODUCTION

The older adult population (defined as those aged 65 years and older) is the fastest growing age group in American society. The US Bureau of the Census reported that in 2010 there were more than 40 million older Americans representing nearly 13% of the population. The Census Bureau projects that more than 20% of American adults

Disclosure: All patients in this article were treated by Dr C. Zahedi and all radiographic and clinical material were provided by Dr C. Zahedi. Dr C. Zahedi is a consultant for Mobile Dental USA.

Department of Periodontics, University of California, Los Angeles (UCLA), Implant Mentoring/ Implant Outreach Institute, 4221 MacArthur Blvd, Newport Beach, CA 92660, USA
E-mail address: info@implantmentoring.com

will be aged 65 years or older by the year 2040. The increase in the elderly population has affected the oldest groups the most. For instance, from the beginning of the twentieth century to the present, there has been an 800% increase in the size of the 65-year-old to 74-year-old age group, but the number of Americans aged 85 years and older has increased by 2500% over the same period.[1–3]

The aging population is bringing with it an increase in the number of teeth lost. As a result, the population in need of treatment of complete edentulism is larger than ever.[4]

Oral handicap of complete edentulism can be defined as the physical state of the jaws following removal of all erupted teeth and the condition of the supporting structures available for reconstructive or replacement therapies. It is the terminal outcome of a multifactorial process involving biological factors and patient-related factors. It represents a huge global health care burden and will continue to do so for the foreseeable future.

The fully edentulous orally handicapped older adult population has been neglected because removable acrylic dentures have been the classic therapy for complete edentulism. These soft tissue–supported prostheses do not treat alveolar bone loss or prevent disuse atrophy or pressure-mediated resorption, which are all germane to edentulism. Therefore, they are only rehabilitative, not therapeutic.[5,6]

To address the oral handicap of complete edentulism, osseointegrated endosseous implants should be used as a therapeutic adjunct. Implants can reduce the problem of long-term bone resorption to less than 0.1 mm per year while providing adequate masticatory function.[7]

However, most denture wearers are not aware that the pressure of their removable dentures on the jaw results in the loss of the jaw bone, thus reducing the stability of their dentures. It can be frustrating to eat certain foods or to try to speak with confidence with the fear that the denture will begin to float in the mouth. Not replacing missing teeth with stable dentures prevents adequate food intake, resulting in a lack of proper nutrients and vitamins and leading to weight loss and serious medical conditions such as heart disease and poor cognitive function.[7–9] A low number of teeth increases the risk of higher prevalence and incidence of dementia.[10]

To address the disease of edentulism, endosseous implants are being used as a therapeutic adjunct and can reduce the problem of long-term bone resorption to less than 0.1 mm per year. Dental implants offer many advantages in the oral rehabilitation of older patients.[11] The use of dental implants for support and/or retention of fixed or removable prostheses has been shown to be an important opportunity to enhance prosthodontic treatment outcomes and quality of life for patients with complete edentulism.[12]

This article reviews and discusses the current techniques to rehabilitate fully edentulous older adult patients by means of dental implants.

OSSEOINTEGRATION

Osseointegration of the implants to the bone is one the most crucial factors that influences the long-term predictability of the implant placement procedure. Osseointegration, defined as a direct structural and functional connection between ordered, living bone and the surface of a load-carrying implant, is critical for implant stability, and is considered a prerequisite for implant loading and long-term clinical success of endosseous dental implants.[13] Osseointegration involves an initial interlocking between alveolar bone and the implant body, and, later, biological fixation through continuous bone apposition and remodeling toward the implant. It is a complex process in which many factors influence the formation and maintenance of bone at the implant surface.[14]

Indications for Dental Implants for Older Adults

There are a myriad of treatment options and related investment (costs) for completely edentulous patients. They range from overdentures supported by only 2 implants to full-arch fixed partial dentures (implant bridges) supported by 4 or more implants.

The indications for dental implants in older adults are in general not different from the rest of the population because chronologic age is not a contraindication for dental implants. It has also been reported that older individuals respond to oral implants in the same manner as younger adults, despite their tendency for systemic illness.[12]

In a comparison of 2 closely matched groups of completely edentulous younger and older patients with dental implants after follow-up times of 4 to 16 years, a cumulative success rate of 92% in the older group and 86.5% in the younger group were reported.[15] Even more importantly, the prosthesis success rate was 100%, and the original prosthesis was in place throughout the respective observation periods for 41 of 45 of the older patients. The remaining prostheses needed repair at some point in the follow-up.[15]

The mental state of edentulous patients can be improved with overdentures and the enhancement can be caused by functional improvement with prostheses when loaded with implants and not by the mere existence of implants without any function.[16]

Precautions for Medically Compromised Patients

Medically compromised patients are defined as patients with decreased or compromised physical and mental ability to perform regular tasks compared with normal people of same age.[17]

Cardiac systemic diseases

Implants in patients with cardiac systemic diseases may show lower levels of osseointegration caused by compromised oxygen and nutrient supply in the bone. These patients may also be at a higher risk of developing infective endocarditis.[18–20] Dentists should take the opinion of the primary physicians of the patients about whether the condition is medically controlled or not.

Radiotherapy

Radiotherapy is not considered a major risk factor for implant loss. However, it might lead to implant loss or negatively affect osseointegration if it is administered over the oral cavity, involves ionizing radiation, or the radiation dose is higher than 50 Gy.[17]

Tobacco

Consumption of tobacco has been significantly associated with implant loss. The implant failure rate is 2.5 to 2.6 times higher in patients who smoke compared with nonsmokers.[21–23]

Diabetes

In the past, type II diabetes was considered an absolute contraindication because of risk of infection and failure of osseointegration, but more recent studies[24,25] have shown that the implant failure rate is much lower if the condition is controlled. The surgery needs to be done using aseptic techniques accompanied by an appropriate antibiotic regimen.

Osteoporosis

Osteoporosis has been considered as a risk factor for implant failure because of the bone loss that occurs in this condition, but most recent studies[23,26–28] have concluded that it should not be considered as a contraindication for implant placement. However, if the patient is taking oral bisphosphonates, the condition should be treated as a relative or partial contraindication. It is an absolute contraindication if bisphosphonates are being delivered intravenously or there is an associated corticosteroid, immune-suppressor, or hormonal therapy regimen.

In conclusion, systemic conditions do not affect implant survival if they are controlled,[29] but this needs to be confirmed with randomized controlled trials. It is more important for the disease to be in a controlled condition than the disease itself and, to determine the appropriate course of action, a proper medical examination needs to be done.[30]

SIMPLIFICATION AND RATIONALIZATION

Several rules, often considered as dogmas, made it possible for oral implants to achieve a high success rate. However, some of these concepts have been questioned. The submerged nature of implant placement, the arbitrary 3-month to 6-month healing period, bicortical anchorage, placement of the longest possible implants, as well as implant placement in strict sterile conditions have been scientifically challenged. An in-depth knowledge and experience in both the surgical and prosthetic aspects of oral implantology are of utmost importance in order to achieve a high success rate.[31]

Types of Dental Implants

There are 3 types of implants, and they can be described according to their shape and how they are attached to the jaw (**Fig. 1**):

1. Endosseous implants are usually shaped like a screw or cylinder and are placed within the jawbone. There are also blade-shaped endosseous implants. Osseointegrated endosseous dental implants have provided successful and predictable long-term results.[32]
2. Subperiosteal implants consist of a metal framework that attaches on top of the jawbone but underneath the gum tissue (**Fig. 2**).
3. Transosteal implants are either a metal pin or a U-shaped frame that passes through the jawbone and the gum tissue, into the mouth.

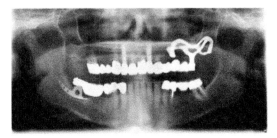

Fig. 1. Panoramic radiograph of an older adult showing on the upper left a subperiosteal implant and on the lower right a blade implant. There are also 2 endosseous screw-type implants on the maxillary anterior.

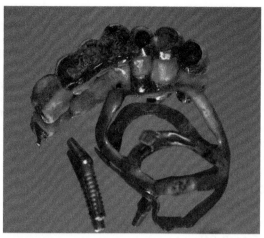

Fig. 2. Patient was complaining for more than 2 years of bad smell and taste in his mouth. The removed subperiosteal implant is shown, along with an endosseous implant after removal of the bridge. Huge amounts of plaque and food debris have accumulated under the bridge.

Bone Regeneration Before or Immediately after Implant Placement

Bone volume (quantity) and density (quality) are the main prerequisites for safe and predictable implant placement and for attaining the functional stability of the implant needed to achieve osseointegration.

The bone morphology at the osteotomy site influences the ideal implant position at placement. Any deficiency in horizontal and vertical dimensions might require bone augmentation procedures.

Animal studies have also shown that guided bone regeneration using membranes is successful to regenerate bone by protecting the blood clot from the surrounding soft tissue.[33–35] Animal studies have shown that bone grafting around implants at insertion is feasible and histologically documented.[36]

Clinically, various bone substitutes for bone grafting have been used successfully in several indications and histologic and clinical outcomes reported in different oral bone regenerative procedures, such as socket preservation, immediate implant placement,[37] sinus grafting, and lateral and vertical bone augmentation.

Each biomaterial has advantages and disadvantages that are discussed in various reviews.[38,39]

FACTORS AFFECTING IMPLANT LOSS

The stabilization of the lower denture with at least 2 endosseous implants has been used for more than 20 years and was already recommended in the McGill consensus statement as standard therapy in 2002.[40,41]

A recent systematic review of factors associated with postloading implant loss in implant-supported prostheses in edentulous jaws analyzed the potential impact of implant location (maxilla vs mandible), implant number per patient, type of prosthesis (removable vs fixed), and type of attachment system (screw retained, ball vs telescopic crown) on implant loss.[42]

The 5-year survival rate of implants was about 98% and it was slightly higher in mandible than maxilla. In contrast, implant loss rate was significantly higher ($P = .05$) in maxilla compared with mandible.

Loss of implants was greater with removable prostheses than with fixed restorations ($P<.05$). The lower the number of implants, the higher the implant loss rate with fixed restorations.[42] Similar results were found with overdentures: the lower the number of implants, the higher the implant loss rate with maxillary and mandibular overdentures. The investigators concluded that the implant location and the number and type of prostheses affect the implant rate. Hence, during treatment planning, the number of implants should be decided by taking into account the type of the prosthesis preferred by the patient and the location of the implants:

RECOMMENDATIONS

Maxilla:
- For removable overdentures: 4 or more implants provide favorable results (see **Fig. 1** and **2**; **Figs. 3–21**)
- For fixed prostheses: 6 or more implants provide good results (**Figs. 22–25**).

Mandible:
- For removable overdentures: 2 or more implants provide favorable results (**Figs. 26–44**)
- Four implants with removable prostheses showed more favorable results than the same number of implants with fixed prosthesis
- For fixed prostheses: 4 or more implants provide good results

Reduced-diameter Implants

A systemic review of the success of narrow-diameter dental implants concluded that narrow-diameter implants of 3.3 to 3.5 mm are well documented in all indications including load-bearing posterior regions. Smaller implants of 3.0 to 3.25 mm in diameter are well documented only for single-tooth non–load-bearing regions. Mini-implants less than 3.0 mm in diameter are only documented for the edentulous arch and single-tooth non–load-bearing regions[43] (**Figs. 45** and **46**).

Mini–dental implants can provide immediate stabilization of a dental prosthetic appliance after a minimally invasive procedure. Furthermore, mini-implants can

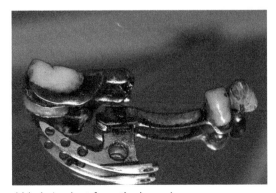

Fig. 3. The removed blade implant from the lower jaw.

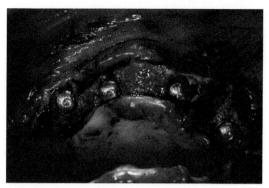

Fig. 4. Four osseointegrated endosseous dental implants inserted in the maxilla.

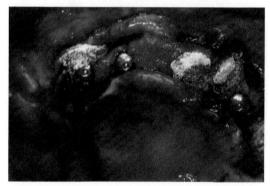

Fig. 5. Bone grafting was necessary because of insufficient bone volume and to preserve the bone volume at the extraction site.

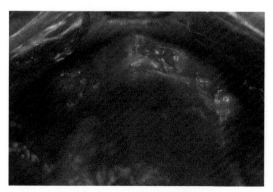

Fig. 6. Soft tissue healing following the placement of implants and bone grafts.

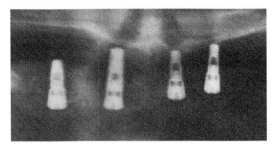

Fig. 7. Panoramic radiographic view following the placement of 4 endosseous osseointe-grated implants.

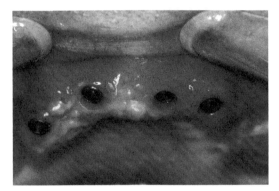

Fig. 8. Soft tissue healing 3 weeks after the second-phase surgery and exposing the implants to the oral cavity.

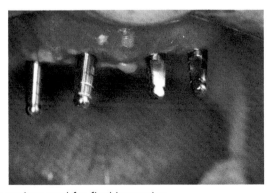

Fig. 9. Impression copings used for final impression.

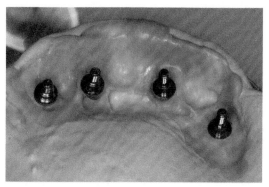

Fig. 10. Impression copings in the final impression.

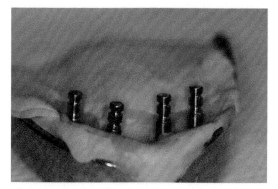

Fig. 11. Implant analogs attached to the impression copings.

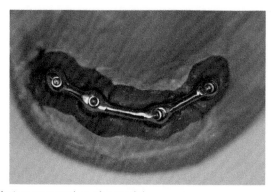

Fig. 12. Cast bar being prepared on the model.

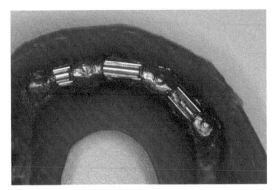

Fig. 13. The overdenture with attachments.

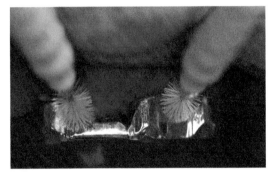

Fig. 14. The patient is instructed on the proper oral hygiene/plaque control methods using appropriate-sized interdental brushes.

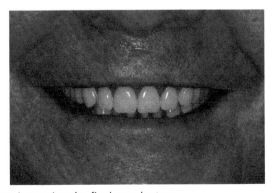

Fig. 15. The patient is wearing the final overdenture.

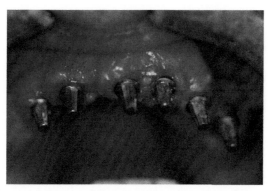

Fig. 16. Six maxillary implants on a fully edentulous older adult patient.

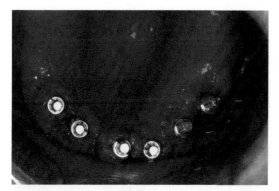

Fig. 17. Occlusal view of the maxillary implants.

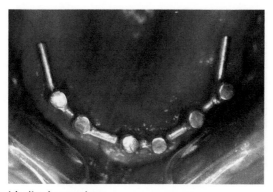

Fig. 18. Cast bar with distal extensions.

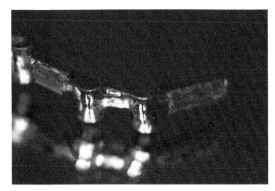

Fig. 19. Attachment connecting the overdenture to the cast bar.

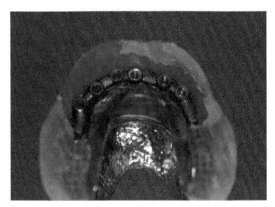

Fig. 20. Cast bar in the overdenture before final connection to the maxillary implants.

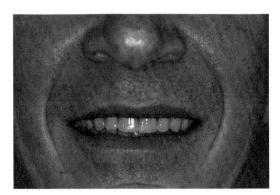

Fig. 21. Final maxillary overdenture.

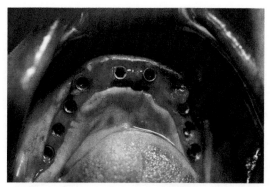

Fig. 22. Intrasurgical occlusal view showing the placement of osseointegrated implants on the mandible for a fixed partial denture (implant bridge).

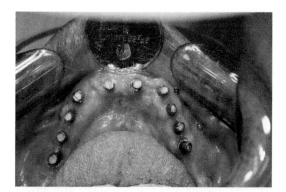

Fig. 23. Occlusal view of the healed soft tissue around the prosthetic abutments.

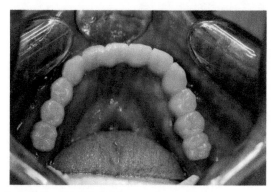

Fig. 24. Occlusal view of the zirconia bridge.

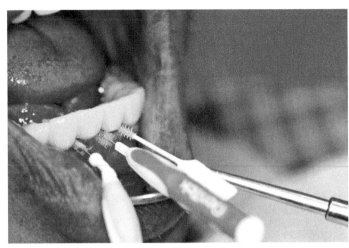

Fig. 25. This older adult has been instructed to use interproximal brushes for optimal plaque control.

be used in cases in which traditional implants are impractical, or when a different type of anchorage system is needed. Healing time required for mini-implant placement is typically shorter than that associated with conventional 2-stage implant placement and the accompanying extensive surgical procedure.

Overdentures retained by 2 to 4 mini-implants can achieve oral health–related quality of life and satisfaction at least comparable with that of 2 standard implants. However, the survival rate of mini-implants is not as high as that of standard implants.[44]

The design of mini-implants is such that insertion techniques minimize peri-implant tissue and bone damage. Because of their versatility and ease of insertion, mini-implants have proved useful as transitional stabilizers and as fixtures for long-term prosthesis function.

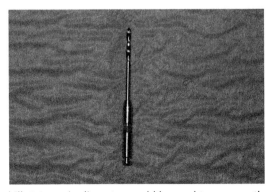

Fig. 26. Only one drill, 1.1 mm in diameter, could be used to prepare the osteotomy site to place mini–dental implants.

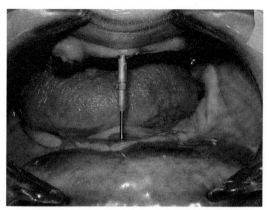

Fig. 27. To place mini-implants, first, a drill is used to locate the midline and the proper mesiodistal and buccolingual direction of insertion. However, in most cases, no mini-implants are placed on the midline. This first drill is only used as a direction indicator.

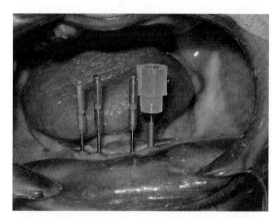

Fig. 28. Once all osteotomy sites are ready, mini-implants are inserted manually.

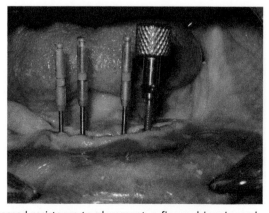

Fig. 29. With increased resistance to placement, a finger driver is used.

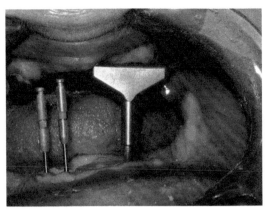

Fig. 30. The finger driver is followed by a winged thumb wrench until the wrench becomes difficult to turn.

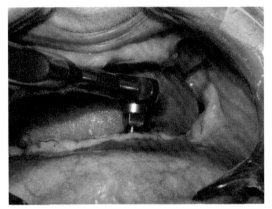

Fig. 31. A ratchet wrench or an adjustable torque wrench then finalizes the insertion process.

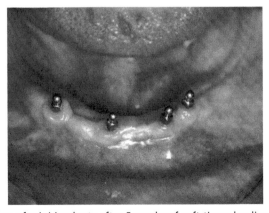

Fig. 32. Buccal view of mini-implants after 3 weeks of soft tissue healing.

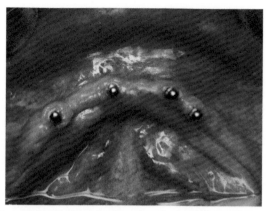

Fig. 33. Occlusal view after soft tissue healing showing a sufficient band of attached kerati-nized mucosa around all 4 mini–dental implants.

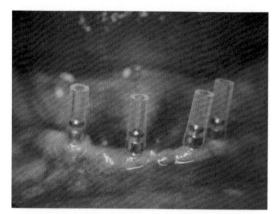

Fig. 34. Blockout shims placed over mini–dental implants to prevent the interlocking of hard acrylic resin after polymerization.

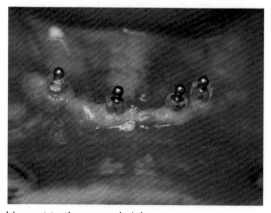

Fig. 35. Blockout shims cut to the proper height.

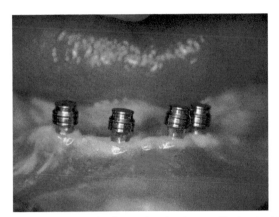

Fig. 36. Metal housings are attached to the implants. Blockout shims are verified individually.

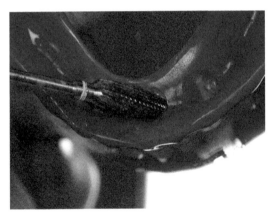

Fig. 37. Relieve the intaglio surface of the denture base at least 1 mm around the metal housings to prevent overload on any single mini-implant.

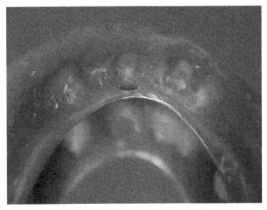

Fig. 38. Sufficient space is created on the intaglio surface of the overdenture to accommodate the metal housings.

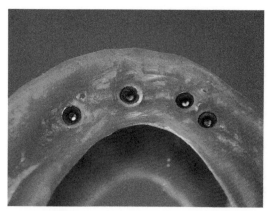

Fig. 39. Metal housings including the O-rings are now connected to the overdenture using acrylic resin.

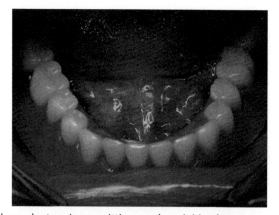

Fig. 40. The final overdenture is now sitting on the mini-implants.

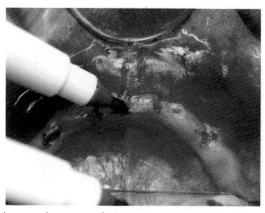

Fig. 41. Using markers on the mucosa for more precise insertion of the drills.

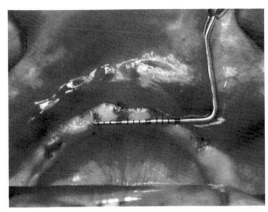

Fig. 42. Measurement of interimplant distances using a 15-mm periodontal proble.

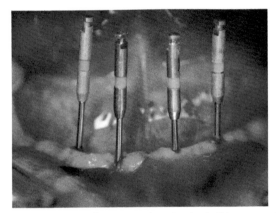

Fig. 43. Guide drills already inserted to ensure interimplant distances and parallelism.

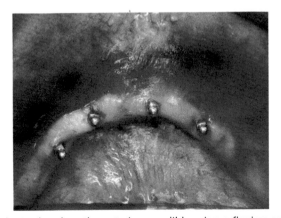

Fig. 44. Mini-implants placed on the anterior mandible using a flapless approach.

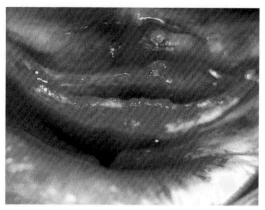

Fig. 45. Very thin ridge on the mandible precluding the placement of regular-diameter implants.

A biometric analysis of 1029 mini dental implant, 5 months to 8 years in vivo, representing 5 clinics, showed a failure rate for stabilization on average of 8.83%, showing fairly consistent long-term prosthesis stabilization and implant success.[45]

Mobile Dental USA specializes in treating older adults in nursing homes and assisted living communities (www.mobiledentalusa.com), and offers a solution called the Bone-loss and Denture-loss Prevention Program™. This solution includes the use of regular-diameter implants but also mini–dental implants. When using mini–dental implants, the Bone-loss and Denture-loss Prevention Program™ offers several advantages:

- Eliminates the life-threatening risk of residents swallowing their removable dentures.
- Improved overall health and increased life expectancy by enabling residents to eat using stable dentures without the need for denture adhesives.

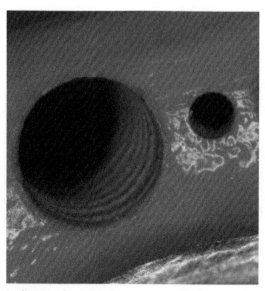

Fig. 46. Difference in diameter between the osteotomy site for a regular-sized (*left*) versus a mini–dental implant (*right*).

- Residents can immediately start eating and speak with confidence.
- Reduced healing time: this is a 1-step procedure that can be done in 1 hour and requires no sutures or the typical months of healing.
- Residents with memory loss (Alzheimer, dementia) will never lose their dentures again and could continuously wear dentures even while sleeping.
- The ongoing loss of the jaw bone stops at the implant sites.
- The more the residents bite on the MDIs, the more they stimulate their jaw bones.
- It is impossible to have any cavities or root canal problems on MDIs.
- It is a solution for residents who cannot have extensive surgery for medical reasons.
- Eliminates the cost of replacing lost removable dentures, especially for memory-impaired adults.
- This therapeutic solution is affordable compared with traditional implant solutions.

Preparation

For fully edentulous older adults, the adequacy of existing removable prostheses has to be assessed in terms of their stability, function, esthetics, and material integrity. In most cases, existing dentures are not satisfactory and a new set has to be made to correctly determine the vertical dimension of occlusion, interarch relationship, and tooth positioning for optimal esthetic, phonetic, and functional effects.

The diagnostic denture setup aids clinicians to a great extent with the assessment if a fixed implant–borne prosthesis is feasible or if a removable approach promises to be more favorable.

The use of volumetric imaging, such as cone beam computed tomography (CBCT), is emerging as a valued aid in planning, placement, and restoration of dental implants.

Radiographic guides could simply be made out of the existing dentures (**Figs. 47** and **48**). These guides could then be used as surgical guides (**Fig. 49**). More sophisticated, but also costly, surgical guides could be made by using

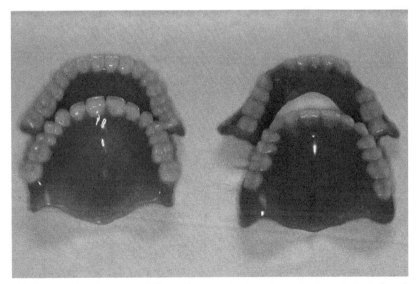

Fig. 47. The existing dentures of the patient can be transformed into radiological and surgical guides.

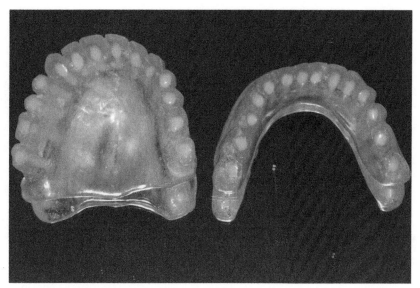

Fig. 48. Radiological guide that will be transformed to a surgical guide after the radiographs (CBCT scans) have been made.

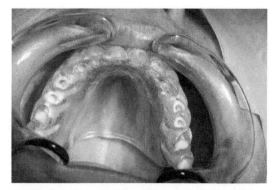

Fig. 49. Surgical guide made by transforming the radiological guide.

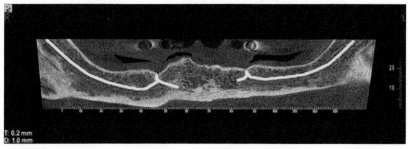

Fig. 50. Two-dimensional (panoramic) view from a CBCT scan on a fully edentulous mandible showing the simulation of the location of the inferior alveolar nerve in yellow.

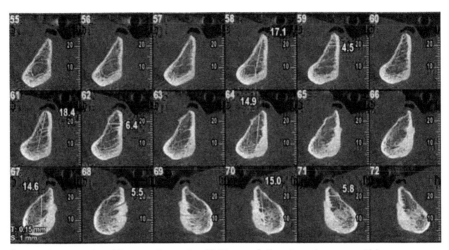

Fig. 51. Cross-sectional images from the CBCT on a fully edentulous mandible.

appropriate software tools that offer three-dimensional control of implant placement.[46]

When using CBCT, clinicians should take into consideration the effective doses for different devices because they have a wide range, with the lowest dose being almost 100 times less than the highest dose.[47] Significant dose reduction can be achieved by adjusting operating parameters, including exposure factors and reducing the field of view to the region of interest[47] (**Figs. 50–52**).

Maintenance

Older adults who have been provided with dental implants should be educated and trained to control plaque biofilm associated with peri-implant tissues and associated restorations.

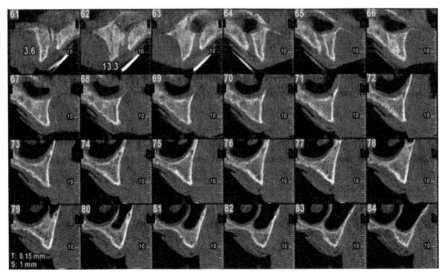

Fig. 52. Cross-sectional images obtained from CBCT showing the limited bone volume in the maxilla.

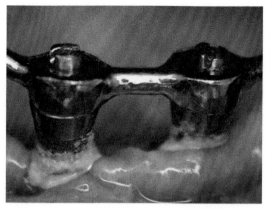

Fig. 53. Insufficient plaque control leading to peri-implant mucositis and peri-implantitis.

There are differences between peri-implant interface and natural teeth that influence the maintenance of soft tissues around implants. The peri-implant soft tissue interface has been shown to be less effective than natural teeth in resisting bacterial invasion. Gingival fiber alignment and reduced vascular supply make the peri-implant soft tissue more vulnerable to subsequent peri-implant disease, such as peri-implant mucositis and peri-implantitis, leading to bone loss around implants.[48] (**Fig. 53**).

Older adult patients with implants should be recalled every 2 to 6 months for examination and professional cleaning. At each visit, ensure that the patient is able to perform optimal plaque removal around the dental implants. Peri-implant tissues should be examined for signs of inflammation and bleeding on probing and/or suppuration and remove supramucosal and submucosal plaque and calculus deposits and excess residual cement. Perform radiographic examination only when clinically indicated.[49]

Implants are probed, examined for stability/mobility, and sites inspected for local disorder (plaque, calculus, bleeding, suppuration) and need for treatment. Assessment of peri-implant mucositis (mucosal inflammation) is primarily made by observing bleeding following light probing (0.25 N) of the implant sulcus/pocket. The absence of bleeding on probing has a high negative predictive value, providing the clinician a predictor of stable peri-implant conditions (**Figs. 54** and **55**).

If inflammation or infection is detected clinically, diagnostic radiographs are obtained as well. Implants become mobile only when advanced bone loss or occlusal

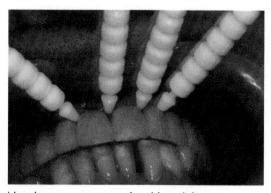

Fig. 54. Interdental brushes are easy to use by older adults.

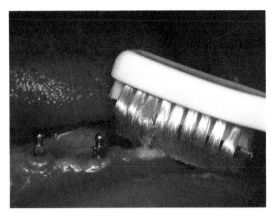

Fig. 55. Special toothbrushes are used around mini-implants.

overload have resulted in the loss of osseointegration. Therefore, the early signs of peri-implant mucositis and peri-implantitis should be diagnosed to provide early treatment.

Implants are in general not instrumented with curettes except for the careful removal of mineralized deposits with special nonmetal curettes, followed by polishing with a nonabrasive or minimally abrasive polishing paste and rubber cup.[50]

REFERENCES

1. He W, Muenchrath MN. 90+ in the United States: 2006–2008 American Community Survey Reports. US Department of Health and Human Services ACS-17. 2011.
2. Doundoulakis JH, Eckert SE, Lindquist CC, et al. The implant-supported overdenture as an alternative to the complete mandibular denture. J Am Dent Assoc 2003;134(11):1455–8.
3. Douglass CW, Shih A, Ostry L. Will there be a need for complete dentures in the United States in 2020? J Prosthet Dent 2002;87(1):5–8.
4. Vos T, Flaxman AD, Naghavi M, et al. Years lived with disability (YLDs) for 1160 sequelae of 289 diseases and injuries 1990-2010: a systematic analysis for the Global Burden of Disease Study 2010. Lancet 2013;380(9859):2163–96.
5. Tallgren A. The continuing reduction of the residual alveolar ridges in complete denture wearers: a mixed-longitudinal study covering 25 years. J Prosthet Dent 1972;27(2):120–32.
6. White GS. Treatment of the edentulous patient. Oral Maxillofac Surg Clin North Am 2015;27(2):265–72.
7. Adell R, Lekholm U, Rockler B, et al. A 15-year study of osseointegrated implants in the treatment of the edentulous jaw. Int J Oral Surg 1981;10(6):387–416.
8. Okamoto N, Morikawa M, Tomioka K, et al. Association between tooth loss and the development of mild memory impairment in the elderly: the Fujiwara-kyo Study. J Alzheimers Dis 2015;44(3):777–86.
9. Liljestrand JM, Havulinna AS, Paju S, et al. Missing teeth predict incident cardiovascular events, diabetes, and death. J Dent Res 2015;94(8):1055–62.
10. Stein PS, Desrosiers M, Donegan SJ, et al. Tooth loss, dementia and neuropathology in the Nun study. J Am Dent Assoc 2007;138(10):1314–22.

11. Feine JS, Carlsson GE. Implant overdentures. The standard of care for edentulous patients. Chicago: Quintessence Publishing; 2003.
12. Bryant SR, Zarb GA. Outcomes of implant prosthodontic treatment in older adults. J Can Dent Assoc 2002;68(2):97–102.
13. Zarb CA, Albrektsson T. Nature of implant attachments. In: Branemark P-I, Zarb C, Albrektsson T, editors. Tissue-integrated prostheses osseointegration in clinical dentistry. Chicago: Quintessence Publishing; 1985. p. 88–98.
14. Albrektsson T, Brånemark PI, Hansson HA, et al. Osseointegrated titanium implants. Requirements for ensuring a long-lasting, direct bone-to-implant anchorage in man. Acta Orthop Scand 1981;52(2):155–70.
15. Bryant SR, Zarb GA. Osseointegration of oral implants in older and younger adults. Int J Oral Maxillofac Implants 1998;13(4):492–9.
16. Banu RF, Veeravalli PT, Kumar VA. Comparative evaluation of changes in brain activity and cognitive function of edentulous patients, with dentures and two-implant supported mandibular overdenture-pilot study. Clin Implant Dent Relat Res 2015. [Epub ahead of print]. http://dx.doi.org/10.1111/cid.12336.
17. Gómez-de Diego R, Mang-de la Rosa M, Romero-Pérez MJ, et al. Indications and contraindications of dental implants in medically compromised patients: update. Med Oral Patol Oral Cir Bucal 2014;19(5):e483–9.
18. Bornstein MM, Cionca N, Mombelli A. Systemic conditions and treatments as risks for implant therapy. Int J Oral Maxillofac Implants 2009;24(Suppl):12–27.
19. Hwang D, Wang HL. Medical contraindications to implant therapy: part II: relative contraindications. Implant Dent 2007;16(1):13–23.
20. Khadivi V, Anderson J, Zarb GA. Cardiovascular disease and treatment outcomes with osseointegration surgery. J Prosthet Dent 1999;81(5):533–6.
21. Wilson TG Jr, Nunn M. The relationship between the interleukin-1 periodontal genotype and implant loss. Initial data. J Periodontol 1999;70(7):724–9.
22. Susarla SM, Chuang SK, Dodson TB. Delayed versus immediate loading of implants: survival analysis and risk factors for dental implant failure. J Oral Maxillofac Surg 2008;66(2):251–5.
23. Holahan CM, Koka S, Kennel KA, et al. Effect of osteoporotic status on the survival of titanium dental implants. Int J Oral Maxillofac Implants 2008;23(5):905–10.
24. Beikler T, Flemmig TF. Implants in the medically compromised patient. Crit Rev Oral Biol Med 2003;14(4):305–16.
25. Morris HF, Ochi S, Winkler S. Implant survival in patients with type 2 diabetes: placement to 36 months. Ann Periodontol 2000;5(1):157–65.
26. Lee JY, Park HJ, Kim JE, et al. A 5-year retrospective clinical study of the Dentium implants. J Adv Prosthodont 2011;3(4):229–35.
27. de Melo L, Piattelli A, Lezzi G, et al. Human histologic evaluation of a six-year-old threaded implant retrieved from a subject with osteoporosis. J Contemp Dent Pract 2008;9(3):99–105.
28. Shibli JA, Aguiar KC, Melo L, et al. Histological comparison between implants retrieved from patients with and without osteoporosis. Int J Oral Maxillofac Surg 2008;37(4):321–7.
29. Lee HJ, Kim YK, Park JY, et al. Short-term clinical retrospective study of implants in geriatric patients older than 70 years. Oral Surg Oral Med Oral Pathol Oral Radiol Endod 2010;110(4):442–6.
30. Diz P, Scully C, Sanz M. Dental implants in the medically compromised patient. J Dent 2013;41(3):195–206.

31. Zahedi CS, Cassin D, Brunel G, et al. Simplification and rationalization of oral implantology. Rev Belge Med Dent 2001;56(1):62–71.
32. Adell R, Eriksson B, Lekholm U, et al. Long-term follow-up study of osseointegrated implants in the treatment of totally edentulous jaws. Int J Oral Maxillofac Implants 1990;5(4):347–59.
33. Zahedi S, Legrand R, Brunel G, et al. Evaluation of a diphenylphosphorylazide-crosslinked collagen membrane for guided bone regeneration in mandibular defects in rats. J Periodontol 1998;69(11):1238–46.
34. Brunel G, Piantoni P, Elharar F, et al. Regeneration of rat calvarial defects using a bioabsorbable membrane technique: influence of collagen cross-linking. J Periodontol 1996;67(12):1342–8.
35. Rompen EH, Biewer R, Vanheusden A, et al. The influence of cortical perforations and of space filling with peripheral blood on the kinetics of guided bone generation. A comparative histometric study in the rat. Clin Oral Implants Res 1999; 10(2):85–94.
36. Alliot B, Piotrowski B, Marin P, et al. Regeneration procedures in immediate transmucosal implants: an animal study. Int J Oral Maxillofac Implants 1999;14(6): 841–8.
37. Benqué E, Zahedi S, Brocard D, et al. Tomodensitometric and histologic evaluation of the combined use of a collagen membrane and a hydroxyapatite spacer for guided bone regeneration: a clinical report. Int J Oral Maxillofac Implants 1999;14(2):258–64.
38. Sanz M, Vignoletti F. Key aspects on the use of bone substitutes for bone regeneration of edentulous ridges. Dent Mater 2015;31(6):640–7.
39. Milinkovic I, Cordaro L. Are there specific indications for the different alveolar bone augmentation procedures for implant placement? A systematic review. Int J Oral Maxillofac Surg 2014;43(5):606–25.
40. Morrow RM, Powell JM, Jameson WS, et al. Tooth-supported complete dentures: description and clinical evaluation of a simplified technique. J Prosthet Dent 1969;22(4):415–24.
41. Feine JS, Carlsson GE, Awad MA, et al. The McGill consensus statement on overdentures. Mandibular two-implant overdentures as first choice standard of care for edentulous patients. Int J Oral Maxillofac Implants 2002;17(4):601–2.
42. Kern JS, Kern T, Wolfart S, et al. A systematic review and meta-analysis of removable and fixed implant-supported prostheses in edentulous jaws: post-loading implant loss. Clin Oral Implants Res 2015;27(2):174–95.
43. Klein MO, Schiegnitz E, Al-Nawas B. Systematic review on success of narrow-diameter dental implants. Int J Oral Maxillofac Implants 2014;29(Suppl):43–54.
44. de Souza RF, Ribeiro AB, Della Vecchia MP, et al. Mini vs. standard implants for mandibular overdentures: a randomized trial. J Dent Res 2015;94(10):1376–84.
45. Bulard RA, Vance JB. Multi-clinic evaluation using mini-dental implants for long-term denture stabilization: a preliminary biometric evaluation. Compend Contin Educ Dent 2005;26(12):892–7.
46. De Kok IJ, Thalji G, Bryington M, et al. Radiographic stents: integrating treatment planning and implant placement. Dent Clin North Am 2014;58(1):181–92.
47. Bornstein MM, Scarfe WC, Vaughn VM, et al. Cone beam computed tomography in implant dentistry: a systematic review focusing on guidelines, indications, and radiation dose risks. Int J Oral Maxillofac Implants 2014;29(Suppl):55–77.
48. Wang Y, Zhang Y, Miron RJ. Health, maintenance, and recovery of soft tissues around implants. Clin Implant Dent Relat Res 2015. [Epub ahead of print].

49. Matthews DC. Prevention and treatment of periodontal diseases in primary care. Evid Based Dent 2014;15(3):68–9.
50. Mishler OP, Shiau HJ. Management of peri-implant disease: a current appraisal. J Evid Based Dent Pract 2014;14(Suppl):53–9.

Communicating with Patients with Special Health Care Needs

Kimberly M. Espinoza, DDS, MPH[a],*, Lisa J. Heaton, PhD[b]

KEYWORDS

- Intellectual disability • Psychiatric conditions • Dental fear
- Communication disorders • Augmentative and alternative communication

KEY POINTS

- Providers should be attentive to the communication needs of patients with special health care needs, including patients with communication disorders, psychiatric conditions, and dental fears.
- Patients with communication disorders have a wide range of communication abilities requiring different levels and types of supports to facilitate communication.
- Providers should have referral sources available for patients in need of additional services for anxiety, depression, or other psychiatric conditions.

Patients with special health care needs (PSCHNs) represent a diverse population of individuals in dental practice. This population includes people who may need additional supports to maintain oral health and access oral health care services, such as those with developmental or acquired disabilities and significant health or mental health conditions. Communication between patients and the health care team is an essential component of accessing quality care. Many PSCHNs face communication challenges in health care settings. These challenges can result in patient frustration, hinder appropriate diagnosis and treatment, and increase the risk of adverse outcomes.[1,2] This article describes communication challenges and how to overcome them when providing care for patients with intellectual disabilities (IDs), communication disorders, dental fears, and psychiatric conditions.

Disclosure: The authors have nothing to disclose.
[a] Dental Education in the Care of Persons with Disabilities Program, Department of Oral Medicine, University of Washington School of Dentistry, 1959 Northeast Pacific Street, Seattle, WA 98195, USA; [b] Department of Oral Health Sciences, University of Washington School of Dentistry, 1959 Northeast Pacific Street, Seattle, WA 98195, USA
* Corresponding author.
E-mail address: kmespino@uw.edu

INTELLECTUAL DISABILITY AND COMMUNICATION DISORDERS

Communication involves the exchange of messages and ideas between individuals and can be divided into receptive communication (receiving, processing, and understanding messages) and expressive communication (planning and producing messages). Communication can be verbal as well as nonverbal, and includes spoken and written messages, sign language, facial expressions, gestures, and body language. Communication disorders for PSHCNs can be caused by cognitive disabilities, speech disorders, and language disorders, as well as impairments affecting vision and hearing. Dental practitioners are likely to encounter patients with communication disorders in their practices. In the United States, there are approximately:

- Three million people with an intellectual disability (ID)
- Seven and a half million with a voice impairment
- Between 6 and 8 million with a language impairment[3,4]

Intellectual Disability

ID is the most common developmental disability and involves deficits in intellectual and adaptive functioning, such as abstract thinking, planning, memory, and interpersonal communication. An ID begins before age 18 years and persists throughout adulthood. Individuals with an ID have a wide range of communication abilities.

Expressive communication

There is considerable variation in the expressive communication abilities of individuals with IDs. Many have strong verbal abilities and discuss their questions and concerns regarding dental care without difficulty. Some use simple phrases or sentences, whereas others are limited to combinations of 1 or 2 word out of a limited vocabulary. Nonverbal messages may be the primary mode of communication and include reaching gestures, such as pointing, as well as body orientation, facial expression, eye gaze, and vocalizations.[5,6] Those with profound ID are less likely to communicate intentionally and more likely to need interpretation of their behaviors, facial expressions, and body language to determine their moods and preferences.

Some difficulties that can arise with expressive communication among patients with ID include:

- Obtaining a medical history: a survey of physicians found that 89% of general practitioners noted difficulty obtaining a medical history from their patients with ID.[7] When previous medical records are available they can help supplement what is gained from a verbal history. Family members and caregivers may also supplement a medical history when appropriate.
- Describing symptoms: some individuals have difficulty describing symptoms, which can complicate medical and dental diagnoses. The typical problem-focused dental examination may need to be more comprehensive to determine the nature of a problem in the case of a nondescript complaint of oral pain.
- Time needed to respond: some individuals with ID need extra time to process and understand messages received. Allowing additional time for patients to respond can be helpful.
- Familiarity of informants: family members and caregivers can be invaluable informants who are able to supply rich medical, dental, and symptom histories. It presents a challenge when high caregiver turnover results in informants with limited knowledge of a patient's history, needs, and preferences.

- Response biases: sometimes expressive language does not correspond with what a patient is thinking or feeling. This situation can complicate assessing symptoms as well as obtaining informed consent. Examples include:
  - Acquiescence (yea-saying): this is a form of response bias in which an individual has a tendency to say "Yes" to all questions. Yea-saying is a learned adaptation that may help the person avoid feeling embarrassed or getting in trouble.[8,9] It is then applied to other situations, such as the dental encounter. Yea-saying may increase when an individual with ID does not understand what was said and is communicating with someone in a position of authority, such as can happen in a patient-provider relationship. **Table 1** presents several strategies for assessing acquiescence.
  - Nay-saying: this is when an individual has a tendency to respond "No" to all questions.[8] This may also be a learned adaptation, such as a means to escape unwanted situations.
  - Suggestibility: some patients with ID easily internalize the statements of others.[8] For example, when asking whether the patient's tooth hurts, an individual who is highly suggestible may hear the phrase and respond, "Yes, my tooth hurts" despite having no previous symptoms.
  - Recency: when options are given to patients, some individuals have a tendency to choose the last (most recent) option mentioned.[9] Varying the order of choices given can help assess the validity of responses.

Table 1
Strategies for assessing acquiescence

Strategy	Examples	Disadvantage
Nonsense questions: asking absurd questions that should have a "No" answer	"Do you brush your teeth 20 times a day?"	Patients may say "Yes" because they think the question is a joke. Patient may have a valid reason to respond "Yes"[8]
Opposite meanings: asking 2 questions with opposite meanings	"Does your tooth hurt?" "Does your tooth feel good?"	In some situations, it is not illogical to answer "Yes" to both[8] (eg, tooth hurts, but feels smooth to the tongue) Wording of opposite question may be confusing
Different formats: asking the same question in different ways	"Does your tooth hurt?" "How does your tooth feel?" (use of visual pain scale)	Patient may have difficulty responding to some formats, depending on communication abilities[8]
Informant checks: asking caregivers or family members to confirm patient's statements	"Has he been brushing his teeth at home?"	Caregiver may incorrectly contradict a true statement made by the patient[8]
Placebo tests: performing placebo tests that should have "No" responses	"Do you feel this?" when dental explorer is near, but does not touch the oral mucosa	Patient may have valid reason to respond "Yes". Example: feels something other than explorer

Data from Finlay WM, Lyons E. Acquiescence in interviews with people who have mental retardation. Mental Retard 2002;40(1):14–29.

Receptive communication

As with expressive communication, receptive communication is highly variable among individuals with ID. In general, there tends to be stronger receptive than expressive communication abilities in this population.[5] Individuals with ID may be able to understand varying levels of abstract or concrete language as well as nonverbal messages.

Challenges with receptive communication for patients with ID may include:

- Understanding health care messages: supplementing verbal instructions with photographs, models, or hands-on demonstrations can improve patient comprehension, as can the use of concrete words and concepts.[5,10] Many patients with ID require more time or multiple repetitions to understand the health care information given. Patients with ID may understand more than they can readily express.
- Use of informants: informants such as caregivers or family members can help elucidate a patient's level of comprehension. However, in the context of an unfamiliar environment, such as a dental office, receptive communication may be hindered and assumptions of comprehension may be incorrect.[5,11]
- Providing informed consent: it is important to assess whether or not each patient understands the risks, benefits, and alternatives of proposed procedures when obtaining informed consent. Some patients can easily give informed consent for most procedures, whereas others need communication supports to facilitate the informed consent process.[10] When informed consent is needed and a patient is not able to understand the treatment options, a surrogate decision maker should be involved. A legal guardian for the patient, or other representative as allowed by law, can help advocate for the patient's best interests.

As described, patients with ID have a wide variety of abilities when it comes to communication in health care settings. The following vignette involves an actual clinical health care communication challenge that involved diagnosis by pulp testing for a patient with ID.

Vignette 1. Pulp testing for a patient with ID

Alexandra (name changed) was a 24-year-old woman with a mild ID. She presented to dental appointments with her mother, who served as her legal guardian. She had a fistula near tooth 27 and was referred to an endodontist. Alexandra told the endodontist "I was told I have an infected tooth." The endodontist completed vitality testing and determined that the tooth was vital, recommending observation only. The endodontist noted that it was not clear whether the responses to the vitality testing were reliable and advised Alexandra and her mother to call with any symptoms. Alexandra returned several months later to the general dental clinic and her mother reported that she had spent the entire night crying after evaluation by the endodontist. Alexandra confirmed that her tooth hurt when asked and the tooth had developed a periapical radiolucency. Her mother was reluctant to return to the endodontist and she did not believe the tooth was infected because there was no cavity on the tooth. She was encouraged to return to the endodontist and the potential causes of tooth necrosis were explained. At her second endodontic consultation, her mother reported that she was no longer having any pain. Tooth 27 again tested vital, with both cold test and electronic pulp testing. Her mother decided not to proceed with endodontic therapy because of the results of the vitality testing and lack of current symptoms.

When she returned to the general dental clinic the fistula was still present. Cold testing was completed and the reliability of her response to cold testing was further evaluated. All teeth in the quadrant tested vital, with normal responses to cold. A placebo cold test was done near the tooth, without touching it. This phantom tooth also tested vital. In addition, Alexandra tended to smile and answer "Yes" to most questions asked by the provider. Her mother agreed to endodontic therapy after discussion of the false responses to cold testing and further discussion of the causes for tooth necrosis. When the pulp chamber was accessed, it was confirmed that the tooth was necrotic. Three years had passed from the initial clinical findings to the completion of the needed dental treatment.

Lessons learned: (1) acquiescence complicated diagnosis and the ability to produce accurate results with pulp testing. (2) A placebo pulp test was an effective and simple way to confirm acquiescence. (3) Multiple communication challenges contributed to the delayed care, including patient-provider communication, health care team communication, and health literacy. (4) Effective communication between providers, the patient, and the guardian was necessary for moving forward with care.

Speech and Language Disorders

Speech and language disorders include dysarthria, apraxia, stuttering, voice disorders, and aphasia. The most common speech disorder, dysarthria, and the most common language disorder, aphasia, are discussed here.

Dysarthria

Dysarthria is a speech disorder that is caused by neurologic impairment of the control of muscle movements involved in the production of speech. Individuals with dysarthria have a variety of clinical presentations that seem to be correlated with specific neurologic lesions. Dysarthria can originate from upper and lower motor neuron (LMN) lesions as well as lesions affecting the extrapyramidal system.

- Spastic dysarthria: bilateral upper motor neuron (UMN) lesions affecting speech result in spastic dysarthria.[12,13] UMNs involved in speech take messages from the cerebral cortex of the brain to the nuclei of the cranial nerves located in the brainstem. Individuals with spastic dysarthria may have slow, imprecise speech movements associated with hypertonia (increased muscle tone) and weakness. Spastic dysarthria can be caused by degenerative conditions, stroke, cerebral palsy, traumatic brain injury, surgical trauma, and demyelinating conditions.[12]
- Flaccid dysarthria: this type of dysarthria is caused by damage to the LMN system. Cranial nerves V, VII, IX, XI, and XII are involved in the motor production of speech, affecting oral, facial, and laryngeal muscles. The LMNs take messages from the nuclei of the cranial nerves to these muscles. The effect of LMN lesions on speech depends on the cranial nerves involved and is often mild, especially with unilateral, localized lesions.[12] Individuals with flaccid dysarthria have hypotonia (reduced muscle tone) and weakness in the affected areas. Causes of flaccid dysarthria include degenerative conditions, surgical trauma, muscular dystrophy, brainstem strokes, myasthenia gravis, infections, tumors, and demyelinating conditions.[12]
- Ataxic dysarthria: ataxic dysarthria has been linked to disorders of the cerebellum, which helps to coordinate movement. This type of dysarthria can result in uncoordinated speech movements, resulting in an irregular speech pattern. Causes of ataxic dysarthria include degenerative conditions, stroke, demyelinating conditions such as multiple sclerosis, tumors, and surgical trauma.[12]
- Hypokinetic dysarthria: this type of dysarthria and the hyperkinetic dysarthrias are associated with disorders affecting the basal ganglia, which help regulate muscle tone and movement. Individuals with hypokinetic dysarthria have a reduced range of speech movements and produce quiet, breathy speech. The most common cause of hypokinetic dysarthria is degenerative disease, specifically Parkinson's disease and parkinsonism. Other causes include stroke, surgical trauma, and infection.[12]

- Hyperkinetic dysarthrias: there are multiple types of hyperkinetic dysarthrias, including dystonia (involuntary movements caused by contractions of opposing muscle groups), chorea (involuntary rapid movements), athetosis (slow, writhing movements), and tics (rapid coordinated movements). The impact on speech varies depending on how speech movements are affected. In most cases the cause of hyperkinetic dysarthria is unknown. Known causes include Huntington's chorea and other degenerative conditions, tardive dyskinesia, and lithium toxicity.[12]
- Mixed dysarthrias: mixed dysarthrias can involve the UMN, LMN, and extrapyramidal systems. The most common mixed dysarthria is caused by amyotrophic lateral sclerosis, a degenerative condition that involves injury to both UMN and LMN systems.[14] Other causes of mixed dysarthria include Parkinson's disease, strokes, demyelinating conditions such as multiple sclerosis, and congenital conditions such as cerebral palsy.[12]

A quiet background, a familiar listener, and contextual cues can improve speech intelligibility of an individual with dysarthria.[15,16] Providers should ensure that patients with dysarthria are not assumed to have an ID because of the presence of a speech disorder.[16] Use of augmentative and alternative communication (ACC) can facilitate communication for this population, especially in severe cases.[17]

Aphasia
Aphasia is a language disorder that can be caused by stroke, traumatic brain injury, or degenerative conditions affecting the language areas of the brain.[18] Aphasia can be divided into fluent and nonfluent categories. Descriptions of the most common types of aphasia are given here:

- Wernicke's aphasia: this is the most common type of fluent aphasia. With fluent aphasia, the individual is able to string words together into sentences, although the sentences do not necessarily make sense. Individuals with Wernicke's aphasia have difficulty understanding spoken and written messages.
- Broca's aphasia: Broca's aphasia is a nonfluent aphasia, and may involve effortful and agrammatical speech. Individuals with Broca's aphasia may understand much of what is being said by others but have difficulty producing the language needed for communication.
- Global aphasia: this is the most severe aphasia, in which expressive and receptive language are both strongly affected. Individuals with global aphasia may not be able to speak or understand verbal or written messages.

There is a wide range of communication abilities among individuals with aphasia and these abilities can strengthen or weaken over time, depending on the cause and extent of the brain injury.[19] Often individuals with aphasia require a communication partner to assist with communication needs and use ACC techniques.

Augmentative and Alternative Communication
AAC may be used by patients who are not able to communicate their needs through verbal messages alone. AAC is useful to people with a wide variety of communication-related conditions.[20] Main categories of AAC include unaided, low-technology, and high-technology communication strategies.

- Unaided AAC: these strategies involve nonverbal communication. Examples include gestures such as pointing, informal sign language (using personalized signs with symbolic meaning), formal sign language, and blinking or hand squeezing to answer "Yes" or "No" questions.[21]

- Low-technology AAC: these techniques include the use of drawing and writing as well as communication boards or books that can be made by hand or purchased. A common type of communication board is an alphabet board used by patients who are able to spell.[17] Orthotic devices or physical prompts can help patients with movement disorders point to desired items on a communication board.[21] Other communication boards include those containing words, phrases, or symbols that patients can select by pointing, gesturing, or using an eye-gaze technique. An eye-gaze board has matching words or symbols on the front and back of the board along with a large opening in the middle of the board. This arrangement allows the communication partner to follow the eye gaze of the communicator as the communicator selects options from the board. Communication books may contain symbols, photographs, phrases, and words that are arranged thematically or autobiographically in ways that make it easier for the patient to access.[22]
- High-technology AAC: this includes any kind of electronic device to aid communication, such as e-mail, voice amplification, or the use of electronic communication boards.[21,23] Speech generating devices produce digitized speech when patients spell or select desired words, symbols, or pictures using touch or eye tracking systems. High-technology AAC devices include those specifically designed for AAC as well as non–ACC-specific devices, such as tablets or laptops with personal photographs or communication software.[24]

Providers should be attentive to nonverbal cues from patients using AAC and become familiar with AAC strategies and patient preferences for AAC use.[25,26] The following vignette involves a patient with severe dysarthria who used various forms of AAC.

Vignette 2. ACC use in a patient with dysarthria

Chris (name changed) was a 53-year-old man with a progressive demyelinating condition that affected his ability to speak. He presented as a new patient to the dental office. On examination it was determined that he needed multiple dental restorations. He used a communication board as well as facial expressions and gestures to communicate his concerns with the dental team. He was told about the planned treatment and that it would take several appointments to complete. Chris wanted the appointment completed in 1 visit and thought that he did not need the recommended treatment. However, Chris thought that he had been rushed, that his questions were unanswered, and left the appointment frustrated. The staff were frustrated as well. The appointment took longer than they expected and they wished they could do more to help Chris communicate.

Chris came back to the office for a consultation appointment. The team spent more time with him and learned more about his preferences for communicating. Chris also let the team know that e-mail worked much better for him than phone calls and requested appointment cards be written on a full sheet of paper in large print so that he could more easily read them. Communication between Chris and the dental team became much easier and more efficient over time. He was able to have his questions answered and completed all necessary dental treatment. He and the team developed strong relationships and the team always looked forward to his visits.

Lessons learned: (1) the dental team thought that they were better able to support Chris once they became familiar with his communication needs and preferences. (2) Initially, more time was needed for adequate communication of a complex treatment plan. (3) Using multiple types of AAC facilitated needed health care communication. (4) Addressing communication needs and preferences was essential for patient satisfaction and improved the dental team's satisfaction as well.

The FRAME Framework

So far this article has focused on descriptions of various communication disorders and how to address communication challenges with specific populations. The FRAME mnemonic serves as an overall framework for providers to address the communication needs of their patients with communication disorders.[27] This framework was designed by speech-language pathologists at the University of Washington, Department of Rehabilitation Medicine. Providers can reference this useful tool in clinical settings. Key strategies of the FRAME framework are listed in **Table 2**.

DENTAL FEAR AND PSYCHIATRIC CONDITIONS

In addition to addressing communication disorders in practice, appropriate communication for PSHCNs includes sensitivity to each patient's mental health conditions and dental fears. Dentists and dental staff frequently treat patients who have some amount of dental fear. Further, many dental patients experience symptoms of depression and anxiety that are not related to dental treatment. Understanding how to communicate with patients who are dentally fearful, generally anxious, or depressed is key for dental providers to provide high-quality care.

Prevalence and Causes of Dental Fear

In the United States, 5% to 10% of adults avoid dental care because of fear, and as many as 75% of US adults experience at least some dental fear.[28,29] Common fears include pain during and after treatment as well as specific procedures like injections, drilling and oral surgery.[30,31] Treating fearful patients is a common source of stress for dental providers, and this stress can be ameliorated by developing skills to manage these patients appropriately.[32] As discussed later, many of the communication skills used with dentally fearful patients can also be used in interactions with patients who are experiencing depression and/or general anxiety.

Table 2 The FRAME framework		
F	Familiarize	Figure out how the patient best communicates before proceeding with the appointment. This process may involve becoming familiar with existing strategies or establishing new strategies
R	Reduce rate	Reduce your speaking rate and ask 1 thing at a time to lessen the communication burden on the patient. Allow extra time for the patient to respond
A	Assist with message construction	Acknowledge what information you have understood from the patient, agree on how to resolve communication breakdowns. Actively assist the patient with communication
M	Mix communication modalities	Incorporate different ways of communicating, such as writing, drawing, gestures, pictures, and eye gaze, to help patients improve both understanding and expression
E	Engage the patient	Engage the patient directly. Use family or caregivers as interpreters when needed. Keep your focus on interacting with the patient to respect the patient's autonomy

Each letter in the FRAME framework represents a key strategy across a range of communication disorders.
From Burns MI, Baylor CR, Morris MA, et al. Training healthcare providers in patient-provider communication: what speech language pathology and medical education can learn from one another. Aphasiology 2012;26(5):683; with permission.

Prevalence of Psychiatric Conditions

A recent study found that approximately 25% of patients in a general dental practice reported having at least 1 psychiatric condition,[33] which is slightly more than the 12-month prevalence of psychiatric conditions in the general population in 2013.[34] In 2005, antidepressants overtook antihypertensive medications as the most commonly prescribed medication in general medical practice.[35] Although dentists are not trained in diagnosing psychiatric conditions, it is important to be prepared to discuss patients' mental status as needed and refer to the appropriate mental health resources.

- Depression/mood disorders: major depressive disorder is a condition within the classification of mood disorders that may involve feeling sad, sleeping and/or eating more or less than usual, feeling hopeless or empty, losing interest in activities that used to be enjoyable, feelings of guilt or worthlessness, and/or thinking about death or suicide. These symptoms are significant enough to interfere with a person's social and/or work life.
- Anxiety disorders: although many patients are nervous or anxious while sitting in the dental chair, some experience anxiety that extends beyond the dental setting and causes problems with the person's social and work life. Anxiety disorders include social phobia (a fear of negative evaluations from other people); panic disorder (a fear of having a panic attack [a sudden, unexpected rush of fear that includes a racing heart and feelings of lightheadedness]) and generalized anxiety disorder (a consistent state of worry about various aspects of the person's life).

Dental Implications of Psychiatric Conditions

Dental providers are in an excellent position to identify changes in a patient's mental status, particularly in patients whom the dental provider sees regularly. Some signs to look for include:

- A noticeable change in mood from one dental visit to the next. For example, a previously friendly and outgoing patient may suddenly become quiet, sullen, or withdrawn.
- A significant change in oral hygiene. Patients who previously had adequate oral home care who develop a mood disorder may stop taking care of their teeth, resulting in a sudden increase in plaque, calculus, caries, and periodontal disease.
- An increase in no-shows or late cancellations. Individuals who experience an increase in depressive or anxious symptoms may find themselves unable to tolerate a dental appointment, or may not be motivated to pursue dental care, leading them to fail to keep appointments.
- Talk that reflects hopelessness about the future. Patients who are depressed may not want to implement an extensive treatment plan. They may say things like, "I don't know if it's even worth it to get that root canal – I don't know if I'll even be here at the end of the year."

Communicating Techniques

Many of the same communication techniques are useful both with patients who are dentally fearful and with those who are depressed or generally anxious.

- Express concern for patients: "I want you to be comfortable here in our office, and want to do whatever I can to help with your feelings of [anxiety, depression, and so forth]."

- Take time to have a discussion: it is difficult to rush through a conversation about dental fear or depression, and patients pick up on the dentist's desire to get this stage out of the way and focus on dental treatment.
- Use a nonjudgmental tone: avoid making statements like, "You're not afraid, are you?" or, "You're not thinking of doing something crazy, right?"
- Normalize the patient's experience without minimizing: often, patients worry that they are the only people who feel depressed or anxious. Having dental providers reassure patients that they are not alone and that many people feel the same way can make the patients feel more comfortable sharing their feelings with their providers.

For patients who are dentally fearful, dental providers may add the following techniques:

- Ask open-ended questions: a simple, "What's the most difficult part of dentistry for you?" can provide a wealth of information.
- Determine how much information is wanted: some patients wish for a detailed, play-by-play description of the procedure. Others prefer to close their eyes, put on headphones, and be completely disconnected from the appointment. Ask patients what kind of information they would like and when (at the start of the appointment or throughout the procedure?).
- Establish hand signals and time structure: many patients are fearful about not having control during the procedure. Agreeing on a hand signal that patients can use to stop the procedure increases this sense of control. Dental providers can increase patients' sense of predictability by establishing a time structure. For example, the dentist may suggest drilling for a count of 5 to start, or to take a break after 5 minutes.

Sensitive Topics

As described earlier, dental providers often treat patients who are experiencing acute problems, such as depression or anxiety. Similarly, patients may be experiencing situations that, although not directly related to dental care, can affect their lives significantly. As noted earlier, dentists are in a unique position to address such issues with patients, and to provide patients with a safe environment in which to discuss their problems.

- Intimate partner/domestic violence: dentists may treat patients who have unexplained bruises or broken teeth, or patients who seem fearful in the presence of a partner (spouse, boyfriend/girlfriend). A question that has been implemented in many primary care settings is, "Are you safe at home?" This question should be asked away from the patient's partner, if the partner attends the appointment.[36]
- Eating disorders: patients with eating disorders may present with erosion on the lingual surfaces of their teeth from vomiting, or may appear thin and complain of being cold. Dentists can bring up their observations to patients and ask what the patients think is happening. As an example, a dentist might say, "I'm noticing that some of the enamel has been worn away on certain surfaces of your teeth. A lot of times, we see this when someone has had acid reflux or has been vomiting over a long period of time. What do you think might be going on with your teeth? Would it be OK if we talked about what might be going on?" Asking permission to discuss possible reasons for the erosion (or other observations) opens up the discussion without accusing the patient or passing judgment.

The key to discussing any sensitive topic, such as those mentioned earlier, is to avoid making any judgments or scolding the patient. If patients disclose that they have been subjected to intimate partner violence, have an eating disorder, or are experiencing another type of problem, it is key for the dentist to approach the problem in a matter-of-fact way. In addition, dentists can use the following approach to open the discussion:

- Express support: the dentist should thank the patient for sharing what is likely a very difficult topic. The patient should know that the dental office is a safe place to discuss this issue. "I want to start out by thanking you for trusting me with this information – I'm sure it's not easy to bring this up. I want you to know that this is a safe place for you to talk about this, and I want to help you in whatever way I can."
- Listen actively: this is different from trying to solve the problem. Instead, dentists should show the patient that they are listening and are not afraid to have this discussion. This approach means asking questions and restating what the patient says. "What I hear you saying is that you've been making yourself throw up after you eat a lot of food, and you've been doing this more and more over the last month. Is that right?"
- Provide resources: every dentist should have a list of resources, pamphlets, information cards, and so forth, that give contact information for a variety of resources (examples are discussed later). Dentists can provide this to patients by saying, "I want to help you find the best resources for what you're going through. Would it be OK for me to give you some information about [a crisis line, mental health provider, and so forth]?"

Referral Information

Dental providers can give their patients referral information so they can access additional services for their depression, anxiety, and so forth. Useful referral information can include:

- The local or national suicide crisis line for patients who are considering taking their lives (National Suicide Prevention Lifeline: 800-273-8255 or www. suicidepreventionlifeline.org).
- The local or national domestic violence crisis line (National Domestic Violence Hotline: 1-800-799-SAFE[7233]).
- A local psychologist, therapist, or mental health center who may be able to work with patients on their depressive or anxious symptoms.

In sum, if a patient shares such concerns with the dentist, the dentist should do whatever is possible to help the patient access resources. Through a supportive, nonjudgmental tone, the dentist can communicate to patients that the dental office is a safe place to share these concerns, and a place through which they can access the resources they need.

SUMMARY

PSHCNs represent a large category of patients who present to dental practices and are a growing and diverse population. Learning communication techniques for patients with IDs, communication disorders, dental fears, and psychiatric conditions can help promote quality health care. In addition to the review provided in this article, providers are encouraged to learn more about policy and advocacy issues relevant to PSHCNs, disability culture, and general cultural competency training that can help improve access to more appropriate and culturally sensitive care for this population.

REFERENCES

1. Bartlett G, Blais R, Tamblyn R, et al. Impact of patient communication problems on the risk of preventable adverse events in acute care settings. CMAJ 2008; 178(12):1555–62.

2. Wullink M, Veldhuijzen W, Lantman-de Valk HM, et al. Doctor-patient communication with people with intellectual disability – a qualitative study. BMC Fam Pract 2009;10:82.

3. Maulik PB. Prevalence of intellectual disability: a meta-analysis of population-based studies. Res Dev Disabil 2011;32(2):419–36.

4. Statistics on voice, speech, and language. National Institute of Deafness and Other Communication Disorders. Available at: http://www.nidcd.nih.gov/health/statistics/vsl/Pages/stats.aspx. Accessed October 24, 2015.

5. Schalick WO, Westbrook C, Young B. Communication with individuals with intellectual disabilities and psychiatric disabilities: a summary of the literature. Ann Arbor, MI: University of Michigan Retirement Research Center; 2012.

6. Cascella PW. Expressive communication strengths of adults with severe to profound intellectual disabilities as reported by group home staff. Commun Disord Q 2005;26(3):156–63.

7. Lennox NG, Diggens JN, Ugoni AM. The general practice care of people with intellectual disability: barriers and solutions. J Intellect Disabil Res 1997;41(5): 380–90.

8. Finlay WM, Lyons E. Acquiescence in interviews with people who have mental retardation. Ment Retard 2002;40(1):14–29.

9. Heal LW, Sigelman CK. Response biases in interviews of individuals with limited mental ability. J Intellect Disabil Res 1995;39(4):331–40.

10. Dye L, Hare D, Hendy S. Factors impacting on the capacity to consent in people with learning disabilities. Tizard Learn Disabil Rev 2003;8(3):11–20.

11. Purcell M, Morris I, McConkey R. Staff perceptions of the communicative competence of adult persons with intellectual disabilities. Br J Dev Disabil 1999; 45(1):16–25.

12. Duffy JR. Motor speech disorders: substrates, differential diagnosis, and management. St Louis (MO): Elsevier Mosby; 2005.

13. Kent RD, Duffy JR, Slama A, et al. Clinicoanatomic studies in dysarthria: review, critique, and directions for research. J Speech Lang Hear Res 2001;44(3): 535–51.

14. Tomick B, Guiloff RJ. Dysarthria in amyotrophic lateral sclerosis: a review. Amyotroph Lateral Scler 2010;11:4–15.

15. Lee Y, Sung JE, Sim H. Effect of listeners' working memory and noise on speech intelligibility in dysarthria. Clin Linguist Phon 2014;28(10):785–95.

16. Fox A, Pring T. The cognitive competence of speakers with acquired dysarthria: judgements by doctors and speech language therapists. Disabil Rehabil 2005; 27(23):1399–403.

17. Yorkston KM, Hanson E, Beukelman DR. Speech supplementation techniques for dysarthria: a systematic review. Technical Report Number 4. Academy of Neurologic Communication Disorders and Sciences; 2011. Available at: http://www.ancds.org/assets/docs/EBP/tr_4_sp_suppl_technical_report.pdf.

18. Yourganov G, Smith KG, Fridriksson J, et al. Predicting aphasia type from brain damage measured with structural MRI. Coretex 2015;73:203–15.

19. Anglade C, Thiel A, Ansaldo AI. The complementary role of the cerebral hemi-spheres in recovery from aphasia after stroke: a critical review of literature. Brain Inj 2014;28(2):138–45.
20. Beukelman DR, Mirenda P. Augmentative & alternative communication: support-ing children & adults with complex communication needs. Baltimore (MD): Paul H Brookes Publishing; 2013.
21. Beukelman DR, Garrett KL, Yorkston KM. Augmentative communication strategies for adults with acute or chronic medical conditions. Baltimore (MD): Paul H Brookes Publishing; 2007.
22. Beukelman DR, Hux K, Dietz A, et al. Using visual scene displays as comm-unication support options for people with chronic, severe aphasia: a summary of AAC research and future directions. Augment Altern Commun 2015;31(3):234–45.
23. Paterson H, Carpenter C. Using different methods to communicate: how adults with severe acquired communication difficulties make decisions about the communication methods they use and how they experience them. Disabil Rehabil 2015;37(17):1522–30.
24. Light J, McNaughton D. The changing face of augmentative and alternative communication: past, present and future challenges. Augment Altern Commun 2012;28(4):197–204.
25. Finke EH, Light J, Kitko L. A systematic review of the effectiveness of nurse communication with patients with complex communication needs with a focus on the use of augmentative and alternative communication. J Clin Nurs 2008;17(16):2102–15.
26. Balandin S, Hemsley B, Sigafoos J, et al. Communicating with nurses: the expe-riences of 10 adults with cerebral palsy and complex communication needs. Appl Nurs Res 2007;20(2):56–62.
27. Burns MI, Baylor CR, Morris MA, et al. Training healthcare providers in patient-provider communication: what speech language pathology and medical educa-tion can learn from one another. Aphasiology 2012;26(5):673–88.
28. Milgrom P, Fiset L, Melnick S, et al. The prevalence and practice management con-sequences of dental fear in a major US city. J Am Dent Assoc 1988;116(6):641–7.
29. Getka EJ, Glass CR. Behavioral and cognitive-behavioral approaches to the reduction of dental anxiety. Behav Ther 1992;23(3):433–48.
30. Armfield JM, Milgrom P. A clinician guide to patients afraid of dental injections and numbness. SAAD Dig 2011;27:33–9.
31. Oosterink FM, de Jongh A, Aartman IH. What are people afraid of during dental treatment? Anxiety-provoking capacity of 67 stimuli characteristic of the dental setting. Eur J Oral Sci 2008;116(1):44–51.
32. Brahm CO, Lundgren JM, Carlsson SG. Dentists' views on fearful patients. Problems and promises. Swed Dent J 2012;36(2):79–89.
33. Giglio JA, Laskin DM. Prevalence of psychiatric disorders in a group if adult patients seeking general dental care. Quintessence Int 2010;41(5):433–7.
34. Any mental illness among adults. National Institutes of Mental Health. Available at: http://www.nimh.nih.gov/health/statistics/prevalence/any-mental-illness-ami-among-adults.shtml. Accessed October 22, 2015.
35. Cherry DK, Woodwell DA, Rechtsteiner EA. National ambulatory medical care survey: 2005 summary. Adv Data 2007;387:1–39.
36. Mehra V, Family Violence Prevention Fund. Culturally competent responses for identifying and responding to domestic violence in dental care settings. J Calif Dent Assoc 2004;32(5):387–95.

Neurologic Diseases in Special Care Patients

Miriam R. Robbins, DDS, MS

KEYWORDS

- Alzheimer disease • Cerebrovascular accidents • Stroke • Parkinson disease
- Multiple sclerosis • Neurologic conditions • Dental management
- Medically complex

KEY POINTS

- Neurologic diseases can have a major impact on functional capacity.
- Patients with neurologic disease require individualized management considerations depending on the extent of impairment.
- This article reviews 4 of the more common and significant neurologic diseases (Alzheimer disease, cerebrovascular accident/stroke, multiple sclerosis, and Parkinson disease) that are likely to present to a dental office and provides suggestions on the dental management of patients with these conditions.

OVERVIEW

Neurologic diseases can have a major impact on functional capacity. Patients with neurologic disease require individualized management considerations depending on the extent of impairment. This article reviews 4 of the more common and significant neurologic diseases (Alzheimer disease, cerebrovascular accident/stroke, multiple sclerosis, and Parkinson disease) that are likely to present to a dental office and provides suggestions on the dental management of patients with these conditions.

General Considerations for All Patients with Neurologic Diseases

- Determine stability and extent of disease
- Communicate in presence of family or caregiver if patient has cognitive changes
  - Determine who is responsible for informed consent
- Determine impact of disease on activities of daily living (ADLs) (**Box 1**).
  - Performing oral hygiene
- Keep patient free of acute disease

Department of Dental Medicine, Winthrop University Hospital, 200 Old Country Road, Suite 460, Mineola, NY 11501, USA
E-mail address: miriam.robbins@gmail.com

Dent Clin N Am 60 (2016) 707–735
http://dx.doi.org/10.1016/j.cden.2016.03.002
0011-8532/16/$ – see front matter © 2016 Elsevier Inc. All rights reserved.

dental.theclinics.com

Box 1
Activities of daily living

(Basic self-care activities essential for independent living)

- Ambulating
- Transferring
  ◦ Ability to get in and out of bed, chair, or on and off a toilet
- Personal hygiene
  ◦ Bathing, grooming, tooth brushing
- Bladder and bowel management
- Dressing
- Self-feeding

Adapted from Longtermcare.gov. Glossary - long-term care information. 2015. Available at: http://longtermcare.gov/the-basics/glossary/#Activities_of_Daily_Living. Accessed November 8, 2015.

- Maintain oral function
- Retain esthetics
- Modify treatment plans to allow for physical imitations
- Provide aggressive prevention plan
  ◦ Enable patient to participate in his or her oral health
    ▪ May require involvement of family member or caregiver
  ◦ Topical fluorides, more frequent recare appointments, modification of oral hygiene techniques

Clinical Considerations for Patients with Neurologic Diseases

- Modifications dependent on amount of physical impairment
- Moderate/severe
  ◦ Short appointments (30–45 minutes)
  ◦ Mid-morning/early afternoon appointments
    ▪ Time with medications taken to control symptoms
- Assess mobility impairment
  ◦ Assistance patient may need getting to and from operatory
  ◦ Assistance in getting in and out of dental chair
  ◦ Any support needed to maintain patient in upright position in chair
- Patients in wheelchairs
  ◦ Determine if patient can transfer from wheel chair to dental chair
    ▪ If yes, then assist as needed
    ▪ If no, treat in wheelchair
- Deficits in protective airway reflexes
  ◦ Semi-supine position
    ▪ 45°
  ◦ Careful suctioning
  ◦ Use rubber dam
  ◦ Judicious use of ultrasonic scalers and air-water syringes
- Difficulty/fatigue keeping mouth open
  ◦ Mouth prop
  ◦ Bite block
  ◦ Give patient breaks as needed

ALZHEIMER DISEASE
Definition and Epidemiology

Dementia is a term that describes a group of symptoms affecting memory, thinking, and social abilities severely enough to interfere with daily life.[1] Alzheimer disease (AD) is an irreversible progressive neurodegenerative condition and the most common form of dementia, accounting for up to 80% of all cases.[2] It is characterized by a progressive decline in cognitive abilities with loss of higher cortical functions, such as memory, judgment, and abstract thought and is ultimately fatal. It is estimated that 44 million people worldwide have AD, with 1 in 9 (5.3 million) Americans older than 65 affected. It is projected that more than 16 million Americans older than 65 will have the disease by 2050.[3,4] Almost two-thirds of Americans with AD are women, and older African American and Hispanic individuals are more likely to develop it. It is the sixth leading cause of death in the United States and the only one in the top 10 that cannot be prevented, cured, or slowed.

The exact etiology of AD is not known but it is believed to be multifactorial, involving several genetic, environmental, and biologic risk factors. Autopsies of the brains of people with AD are characterized by neuronal loss and the presence of senile plaques, which contain β-amyloid (Aβ) protein and neurofibrillary tangles of hyper-phosphorylated tau protein in the hippocampus.[5] Inflammatory-related proteins have been shown to be involved in the generation of Aβ and tangle formation.[6]

Clinical Presentation

The cognitive changes of AD worsen over time, although the rate of progression is variable. On average, a person with AD lives 4 to 8 years after diagnosis, but often symptoms are present well before a formal diagnosis is made. There is no one laboratory or imaging test to determine if a person has AD. Diagnosis is made on the basis of a history of pattern of symptoms over time, including a clinical history of progressive dementia and the exclusion of other causes (**Box 2**). In addition to changes in cognitive abilities, 90% of people with moderate-to-severe AD manifest with at least one behavioral or psychiatric symptom due to the alteration in processing, integrating, and retrieving new information. Depression, hallucinations, delusions, aggression, agitation, and wandering are all common.

According to the Alzheimer's Association, the following are 10 common warning signs of AD[7]:

- Memory changes that disrupt daily life
- Challenges in planning or solving problems
- Difficulty in completing familiar tasks
- Confusion with time and place
- Trouble understanding visual images and spatial relationships
- Problems with speaking/writing
- Misplacing things
- Decreased/poor judgment
- Withdrawal from work/social activities
- Changes in mood/personality

AD can be separated into 3 different categories: mild (or predementia), moderate, and severe. The Global Deterioration Scale[8] (GDS) further divides the disease into 7 stages and is often used to provide an overview for the stages of cognitive function that can be expected at each phase. It may be difficult to place a person in a specific

> **Box 2**
> **Diagnostic criteria for Alzheimer disease (AD)**
>
> - Insidious and worsening changes in cognitive of neuropsychiatric symptoms that
>   - Interfere with ability to perform usual activities
>   - Represent a decline from previous levels of function
>   - Are not explained by recent stroke, delirium, active neurologic disease, non-neurologic medical comorbidity, major psychiatric disorder, or use of medication with substantial effect on cognition
>
> - Amnestic presentation
>   - Impaired ability to acquire and remember new information
>   - Impaired reasoning and handling of complex tasks
>   - Inability to plan complex or sequential activities
>
> - Nonamnestic
>   - Impaired visuospatial abilities
>   - Object agnosia
>   - Impaired facial recognition
>   - Impaired language function
>   - Aphasia
>   - Changes in personality or behavior
>   - Agitation, impaired motivation, social withdrawal, loss of empathy, compulsive or obsessive behaviors, socially unacceptable behavior
>   - Executive dysfunction
>   - Poor judgment
>   - Poor understanding of safety risks
>
> *Data from* McKhann GM, Knopman DS, Chertkow H, et al. The diagnosis of dementia due to Alzheimer's disease: recommendations from the National Institute on Aging-Alzheimer's Association workgroups on diagnostic guidelines for Alzheimer's disease. Alzheimers Dement 2011;7(3):263–9.

stage due to variable progression of symptoms and overlap. Although the progression of the disease cannot yet be stopped or reversed, early diagnosis is important to allow a patient and their family to plan for the future.

Alzheimer Stages

Mild (pre-dementia)
Stage 1
- No impairment, no memory problems, not detectable[9,10]

Stage 2: Very mild decline (age-associated memory impairment)
- Minor memory deficits
  - Forgetting location of familiar object
  - Forgetting names or dates and later remembering
- No objective evidence of memory deficit during tests
- No deficits in employment or social interaction
- Unlikely to be detected during medical examination or by family/friends

Stage 3: Mild cognitive impairment
- Memory and cognition affected
- Compromised ability to perform complex occupational and social tasks
- Trouble with familiar tasks
- Shortened attention span
- Difficulties in concentration
- Errors in judgment

- Changes in personality
  - May begin to exhibit anxiety
- Upset with new situations

Moderate

Stage 4: Moderate cognitive decline (mean duration 2 years)
- Additional cognitive losses
- Impaired short-term memory
- May forget some personal details
- Difficulty in performing complex activities of daily life
  - Inability to manage finance or pay bills
  - Prepare meals for guest
  - Food shopping
- Flattening of affect and lessening of emotional response

Stage 5: Moderately severe cognitive decline (mean duration 1.5 years)
- Significant confusion
- Incipient deficits in basic day-to-day activities
- Difficulty dressing properly for season or occasion
- Temporal and conceptual confusion
- Agitation, hostility, uncooperativeness, or aggression
- Can usually still bathe and toilet independently
- Still recognize family members and retain some details about personal history, especially their childhood

Late

Stage 6: Severe cognitive decline (mean duration 2.5 years)
- Decreased awareness of environment or surroundings
- Apathy, disorientation
- Major behavioral and psychiatric symptoms
  - Aggressive or violent behavior and delusions common
  - Purposeless, repetitive, or compulsive movements
- Need assistance for most ADLs
- Urinary and fecal incontinence
- Inability to recognize faces
- Inability to remember details of personal history
- Ability to articulate decreases

Stage 7: Very severe cognitive decline
- Constant assistance
- Lost ability to
  - Respond to environment
  - Speak intelligibly
  - Ambulate independently
  - Sit up without support
  - Hold head up
  - Swallow
  - Smile
- Emergence of infantile or primitive reflexes
- Muscle rigidity and limb contractures
- Death

Medical Management

There are currently no medications to cure or definitively stop the progression of AD but there are 2 types of medication approved to lessen the progression of the cognitive symptoms for a limited time (**Box 3**). Early-stage to moderate-stage AD is treated using cholinesterase inhibitors, which prevent the breakdown of acetylcholine and can delay worsening of symptoms for 6 to 12 months for approximately 50% of the patients who take them. Common side effects include gastrointestinal distress (nausea, vomiting, and diarrhea) and dizziness and fatigue. In more advanced disease, an N-methyl D aspartate (NMDA) antagonist (memantine) either alone or with

---

Box 3
Medications commonly used in the treatment of AD

Medication to lessen the progression of AD

Cholinesterase inhibitors

- Galantamine
  - Reminyl
  - Razadyne

- Rivastigmine
  - Exelon

- Donepezil
  - Aricept

- Tacrine
  - Cognex

N-methyl D aspartate (NMDA) antagonist

- Memantine
  - Namenda
  - Axura

Combination of memantine and donepezil

- Namzaric

Medication to treat the behavioral symptoms of AD

- Antidepressants
  - Citalopram (Celexa)
  - Fluoxetine (Prozac)
  - Paroxetine (Paxil)
  - Sertraline (Zoloft)
  - Trazodone (Desyrel)

- Anxiolytics
  - Lorazepam (Ativan)
  - Oxazepam (Serax)
  - Alprazolam (Xanax)
  - Buspirone (BuSpar)

- Antipsychotics
  - Aripiprazole (Abilify)
  - Clozapine (Clozaril)
  - Haloperidol (Haldol)
  - Olanzapine (Zyprexa)
  - Quetiapine (Seroquel)
  - Risperidone (Risperdal)
  - Ziprasidone (Geodon)

donepezil may temporarily delay worsening of symptoms. Additionally, patients will often be on psychotropic medications aimed at controlling behavioral symptoms.[11] These drugs all cause some degree of xerostomia, which can increase the rate of caries and periodontal disease. The antipsychotic medications (especially haloperidol) increase the risk of development of involuntary jaw movements (tardive dyskinesia) that can lead to tooth wear and fracture, difficulty with maintaining removable prostheses, and intraoral trauma secondary to tongue and cheek biting.[12]

Dental Management

Oral health care considerations

- Older adults with AD experience more oral diseases than patients without dementia
  - Significantly increased rates of tooth decay, missing teeth, and periodontal disease[13]
  - Periodontal disease may be implemented in the development and rate of progression of AD[14,15]
  - Oral hygiene becomes compromised as the neurologic degeneration progresses[16,17]
    - ADLs are disrupted by temporal and spatial disorientation and reduced motor skills
    - Patients may forget to remove dental prostheses for cleaning for extended periods of time
    - Oral care may not be high on caregiver's priority list
      - Patients may become resistive or combative
  - Decreased saliva leads to increased cervical caries, gingivitis, and periodontal disease
    - Are medication induced and as a direct result of AD[18]
  - Patients may not be able to communicate that they are experiencing tooth pain
    - Ask caregivers about any recent behavioral changes, including rubbing face or mouth, refusal to eat (especially hard or cold foods) or allow tooth-brushing, or aggressive behavior.

Dental treatment planning must be designed with consideration of the progressive nature of the disease and anticipation of future oral decline.

- Ideally, a care plan should be established as early as possible following a diagnosis that involves family members and/or caregivers
  - Initiate an aggressive prevention plan early
  - Discuss need for assistance and strategies for daily oral care
  - Modifications of technique
- Establish who is responsible for giving informed consent
  - Patient should be given opportunity to take part in decisions about treatment if possible; however, consent for irreversible procedures must be obtained by the patient's legal guardian/power of attorney
- Encourage self-care for as long as possible

Patient Management

- Patients will have good days/bad days
  - May be restless, agitated, or hostile
  - Exhibit generalized agitation and anxiety
- Short morning appointments

- Keep waiting time short
- Decrease environmental stimulus
  - Quiet room, keep music low, turn off intercoms
- Keep family member/caregiver in room
  - Can have hold hands if needed
- Use a calm, gentle, matter-of-fact approach and conversational tone
- Interact with patient calmly
- Use direct eye contact
- Nonverbal communication
  - Facial expressions and body posture important
  - Limit use of face mask
  - Smile, touch patient gently on arm
- Speak slowly and clearly
- Use short words and simple sentences
- Ask one question at a time
  - Yes or No answers
- Offer continuous reassurance as procedure progresses

Treatment Modifications

- Establish a preventive program as soon as possible after diagnosis[19-21]
  - Aimed at maintaining oral health and reducing risk of infection
- Try to save natural teeth and avoid removable prostheses
- Restoration of key teeth
- Patients on antipsychotic medications
  - Monitor for tardive dyskinesia
- Medication-induced xerostomia and high carbohydrate diet
  - Aggressive prevention with fluorides
- More frequent recare appointments
- Caregivers responsible for oral hygiene
  - Educate and reinforce at every visit
  - Oral and written instructions

Early stage

- Routine dental care with minor modifications
- Treatment plans anticipating that patient will eventually not be able to care for teeth
  - Identify key teeth and restore
- Avoid advanced restorative
- Crowns, bridges, implants
- More aggressive prevention
  - Stress importance of preventive oral hygiene
  - Educate family member/caregiver as well
  - Use electric toothbrushes and irrigation aids
- Make use of memory aids to help with oral hygiene
  - Pictures, instruction lists, audio aides

Moderate stage

- Resistant behavior common
  - May be able to do simple restorative
- Focus changes from restorative to prevention

- ○ Careful examination to eliminate any sources of pain or potential infection
- ○ Hand scale instead of using ultrasonic
- Use mouth prop or bite block
- Treat in semisupine position
  - ○ Increased dysphagia and aspiration risk
- Education and reinforcement
  - ○ Caregivers must be involved in oral hygiene
- Minimal changes
  - ○ Reline rather than remake dentures
  - ○ If making new dentures, use old ones to recreate overall shape and tongue space
- More frequent recare appointments
  - ○ Fluoride varnish application at every visit
- May need to consider sedation or general anesthesia if extensive work is needed

Late stage

- Patient may become unmanageable
- Emphasis on maintaining oral comfort and adequate nutritional intake
- Provision of emergency care
- Focus on pain/infection
  - ○ May leave root tips if nonsymptomatic
- Intravenous sedation/general anesthesia may be necessary

CEREBROVASCULAR ACCIDENT (STROKE)
Description and Epidemiology

Cerebrovascular accident (CVA) or stroke is an acute neurologic event caused by a sudden focal interruption of blood supply to a portion of the brain either by ischemia or hemorrhage. The resulting loss of oxygen leads to tissue necrosis in the part of the brain affected and can range from mild to severe neurologic deficits or death. Recently, the term acute stroke has been replaced by the term "brain attack," indicating that it is a medical emergency (similar to a heart attack) that requires immediate intervention aimed at preventing and even reversing permanent damage.

Ischemic strokes (87% of all events) are caused by blockage either from the formation of a thrombus in cerebral blood vessel or occlusion of the vessel by an embolus. Hemorrhagic strokes resulting from vascular rupture make up the remaining 13% and are associated with a higher rate of mortality than ischemic ones. A transient ischemic attack (TIA or ministroke) is characterized by acute loss of focal cerebral function with symptoms that resolve within minutes to hours without any permanent damage as a result of temporary ischemia. Up to 40% of all patients who experience a TIA have a stroke within the year, with 50% occurring within the first 2 days after a TIA.[22]

Stroke is the third most common cause of death in developed countries and the leading cause of serious long-term disability in the United States. Every year

- More than 795,000 people in the United States have a stroke
  - ○ Approximately 610,000 of these are first or new strokes
  - ○ 1 in 4 are in people who have had a previous stroke
- 1 of every 20 deaths (approximately 140,000 Americans per year) is stroke related
- The incidence of TIA is 350,000 annually in the United States[23,24]

Overall, 25% of all patients experiencing stroke die within 1 year of the event. Mortality rates are related to the type of stroke, ranging from 8% for patients experiencing an ischemic stroke to 47% for those undergoing a hemorrhagic event. Of those who survive, 10% recover with no significant neurologic deficit, 50% will have a residual deficit but retain functional independence, and 40% will become disabled, often requiring assistance in ADLs.

Nonmodifiable risk factors for stroke include age, gender, race, ethnicity, and heredity. The chance of stroke doubles for each decade after the age of 55. African American and Native American individuals have a much higher risk of death from a stroke. The stroke risk is greater if there is a family history among first-degree relatives. Men are more likely to have a stroke than women up to 75 years of age, but women have a higher lifetime risk of stroke and are at higher risk of death as a result. Prior history of a stroke, TIA, or myocardial infarction also increases the risk of second event.[25,26]

The most common modifiable risk factor for both ischemic and hemorrhagic stroke is hypertension. Other risk factors that can be changed, treated, or controlled include cigarette smoking, diabetes mellitus, carotid and peripheral artery disease, atrial fibrillation, coronary heart disease, heart failure, hyperlipidemia, obesity, alcohol intake, high fat diet, lack of physical inactivity, and periodontal disease (**Table 1**).[27–29]

Clinical Presentation

Stroke is considered a medical emergency that requires immediate attention. Timely recognition is essential to reduce related morbidity and mortality.[30]

Symptoms of a stroke depend on the area of the brain affected. The following are the 5 major signs of stroke[31]:

- Sudden numbness or weakness of face, arm, or leg, especially on one side of the body
- Sudden confusion or trouble speaking or understanding speech
- Sudden trouble seeing in one or both eyes
- Sudden trouble walking, dizziness, or loss of balance or coordination
- Sudden severe headache with no known cause

The degree of residual deficit is dependent on location in the brain and extent of tissue damage that occurs and can include dysphasia and aphasia, hemiplegia or

Table 1 Risk factors for stroke	
Nonmodifiable Risk Factors	**Modifiable/Treatable Risk Factors**
Age of patient	Hypertension
>65	Previous cardiovascular accident
Gender	Previous myocardial infarction
Men > women up to 75	Coronary heart disease
Women > men >75	Carotid and peripheral artery disease
Race	Atrial fibrillation
African American	Congestive heart failure
Heredity	Hyperlipidemia
Family history	Diabetes
	Smoking
	Obesity
	Sedentary lifestyle
	Excessive alcohol intake
	Poor diet
	Oral contraceptive use
	Stress
	Periodontal disease

hemiparesis, apraxia, loss of balance or coordination, and memory and cognitive changes.

Medical Management

The best treatment for stroke is prevention. Control of all modifiable risk factors plays an essential role in reducing the incidence of stroke, with blood pressure control the most important factor. Reduction of systolic pressure by 10 mm Hg can reduce the risk of stroke by 30% to 40%.[32] Tobacco cessation, exercise, eating a low fat diet, and controlling diabetes and cholesterol are also important in prevention. Medications including antithrombotics aimed at decreasing platelet aggregation (including aspirin) and cholesterol-lowering drugs such as statins can reduce stroke risk up to 25%.[33,34]

Early diagnosis and treatment are critical. The phrase "time is brain" emphasizes that human nervous tissue is rapidly lost as stroke progresses and emergent evaluation and therapy are required.[35] Provision of basic life support and activation of emergency response system as quickly as possible will allow the transportation of the patient to a medical center where laboratory and diagnostic testing can be performed to determine if a stroke has occurred. Computed tomography scan can be used to see if the stroke is due to bleeding or occlusion and help determine management aimed at either preventing further thrombosis or hemorrhage. In the case of thrombo-emboli, rapid thrombolysis by administration of intravenous recombinant tissue-type plasminogen activator (rt-PA) within 3 hours of the onset of symptoms improves the chances of recovery.[36,37] Another treatment option is an endovascular procedure called mechanical thrombectomy, in which the clot is removed via a catheter threaded through the femoral artery to the site of the blocked blood vessel in the brain.[38] Endovascular procedures can also be used in certain hemorrhagic strokes by using the catheter to deposit a coil or clip at the site of rupture.[39,40]

In the case of an ischemic stroke, once the patient has been stabilized, medications are administered to reduce the risk of another stroke (antithrombotics, statins, and antihypertensive drugs) and the patient begins the process of rehabilitation. Neurologic recovery depends on the extent and location of brain injury, whether early treatment was done, and the patient's prestroke baseline. Neurologic recovery (regaining lost abilities) occurs in the first few months after a stroke. Functional recovery (improvements in day-to-day functions) can take up to a year. Both involve a multidisciplinary approach involving physical, occupational, and speech therapy depending on the neurologic deficits that have occurred. Even with intense rehabilitation, many patients are left with some degree of permanent disability.[41,42]

Dental Management

Issues to be considered when treating patients at risk for or after a stroke include screening for risk factors, medication-induced coagulation issues, potential drug interactions, stress that might be precipitated by dental care, presence of physical disabilities including communication issues, and the need for individualized oral care plans.

Dentists should identify stroke-prone patients such as older patients with history of hypertension, cardiovascular disease, diabetes mellitus, smoking, previous stroke, TIA, or myocardial infarction. Blood pressure measurement should be done routinely at the initial visit, at all recare appointments, and before any surgical procedure. Patients with risk factors should be encouraged to seek medical care and control or eliminate all possible factors.

In addition to traditional risk factors, the presence of carotid calcifications seen on routine panoramic radiographs (near the angle of the mandible) may indicate an increased risk for stroke and warrants referral to the patient's physician for further evaluation.[27,43]

Initial evaluation of patients with history of TIA or stroke should include the date of the event, underlying comorbidities, current status, medical management, and residual disabilities. Thirty percent of ischemic recurrences occur within the first month following a stroke and the risk of recurrence remains high for the first 6 months, therefore deferral of elective dental care is advised during this period. Patients who have recently experienced a TIA should be considered clinically unstable and also should not undergo dental treatment without medical consultation first.[44,45]

Initial Visit

- Obtain thorough medical history
- Identify at-risk patients
  - Hypertension, diabetes mellitus, cardiac arrest, elevated cholesterol, smoking, TIA or previous stroke, age
- Carotid calcifications on panoramic radiographs[43]
- Document and monitor blood pressure and pulse
- Encourage control of modifiable risk factors
- Patients with TIA
  - Less than 1 month
    - Unstable, no elective care
  - Use caution for first 3 months
- History of stroke
  - Use caution for first 6 months, defer elective treatment
  - Monitor blood pressure and pulse at every visit
- Evaluate physical limitations
  - Hemiplegia, hemiparesis, paralysis
- Impaired mastication and nutrition risk factors
- Determine mobility and ability to get to operatory
- Make sure to clear all obstacles out of way
- Assist as needed

Patients will be taking antiplatelet or anticoagulation medications, increasing the risk of bleeding (**Box 4**). Data indicate that alteration in these regimens for dental treatment increases the risk of adverse events. Therefore, it is not advisable to discontinue these medications before treatment. There is currently no clinically relevant test to measure the degree of anticoagulation for patients taking the novel oral anticoagulant agents (direct thrombin inhibitors and factor Xa inhibitors) or antiplatelet medications. Single/combination antiplatelet medications usually do not cause bleeding of clinical significance that cannot be controlled locally. The novel oral anticoagulants appear to produce similar degrees of bleeding. For patients on warfarin, an international normalized ratio (INR) level of less than 3.5 is acceptable for most dental procedures, including surgery. If the INR is greater than 3.5, then the physician should be consulted with the goal of reducing the dose of warfarin rather than discontinuing it so as to minimize significant adverse outcomes. Local measures including pressure, primary closure, and topical hemostatic agents are usually sufficient to control bleeding.[46]

A stroke can have profound effects on the oral structures, resulting in difficulties in swallowing, eating, and communication (**Box 5**). Loss of the swallow reflex and dysphagia occurs in up to 50% of all patients,[47] leading to increased potential for aspiration. Unilateral damage to the motor nerve supply to the face can result in loss of

---

Box 4
Medications that increase bleeding

- Antiplatelet therapy
  - No clinically relevant laboratory test available
  - Do not discontinue for routine dental procedures, including surgery
  - Use local measures to minimize hemorrhage
    - Atraumatic technique, pressure, 1° closure, topical hemostatic agents
- Dual therapy (eg, aspirin and clopidogrel)
  - If extent of surgery warrants, discuss with physician discontinuing clopidogrel 3 days preoperative and continue aspirin
- Anticoagulation therapy
  - Warfarin
    - International normalized ratio (INR) before invasive procedures
      - INR less than 3.5
        - Treat without modification of dosage
      - INR greater than 3.5
        - Consult with physician to lower dose instead of discontinuing
    - Use local measures to control bleeding
  - Novel anticoagulants (direct thrombin inhibitor/Factor Xa inhibitor)
    - No clinically relevant laboratory test available
    - Do not discontinue for routine dental procedures
    - Use local measures to control bleeding

---

voluntary muscle movement with associated problems of speech. Lack of muscle tone of the tongue on the affected side can lead to decreased ability to self-cleanse the oral cavity, and accumulation of food and debris in the buccal vestibules leads to increased decay. Patients may neglect the affected side of the body and brush only the unaffected side.

The patient's cognitive level and ability to communicate should be established. When speaking to the patient, practitioners should stand facing the patient's unaffected side at eye level without a mask. Different communication techniques may be necessary depending on whether the patient experienced a left-sided or right-sided stroke (**Box 6**). Short, mid-morning appointments are recommended. Patients

---

Box 5
Oral manifestations of stroke

- Motor impairment affects speech, mastication, and swallowing

- Paralysis of soft palate
  - Decreased airway protection
  - Dysphonia

- Unilateral paralysis/flaccidity of orofacial musculature
  - Dysphagia

- Loss of sensory stimuli
  - Unable to chew properly or form bolus
  - Poor lip seal

- Deviation of tongue to side of deficit

- Unable to self-cleanse oral cavity on affected side
  - Increased food and debris around teeth and in vestibule

Box 6
Communication with patient after stroke

Right-Sided Cerebrovascular Accident (CVA) (Affects the Left Side of the Body)

- Difficulty with spatial-perceptual tasks
  - Stand on patient's right side
  - Avoid sudden gestures
- Impulsive and overconfident
  - May deny deficits
- Difficulty sequencing tasks
  - Break tasks into simple steps
- Short attention span
- Learns best by verbal instructions
  - Frequent verbal feedback
- Have patient demonstrate instructions by talking thorough task

Left-sided CVA (Affects the Right Side of the Body)

- Language and speech problems
  - Establish ability to communicate
    - May need to communicate with family or caregiver as well
  - Reading comprehension may also be impaired
    - Consent forms, postoperative instructions
- Speak in short simple sentences
  - Ask yes/no questions
- Face patient without mask
- Decreased auditory memory
  - Demonstration rather than verbal instruction
  - Use drawings to explain procedures

Adapted from Little JW, Falace DA, Miller CS, Rhodus NL. Neurologic disorders. In: Little JW, Falace DA, Miller CS, et al, editors. Little and Falace's dental management of the medically compromised patient. 8th edition. Mosby; 2013. p. 503; and American Stroke Association. Available at: http://www.strokeassociation.org/STROKEORG/AboutStroke/EffectsofStroke/Effects-of-Stroke_UCM_308534_SubHomePage.jsp. Accessed October 29, 2015.

---

may require assistance getting to the operatory and transferring to the dental chair. Blood pressure and pulse should be checked at each appointment. Appointments should be kept as stress free as possible. Good pain control is essential and limited local anesthesia with epinephrine should be used to ensure profound anesthesia. Careful chair position and suctioning should be used in patients with impaired swallowing.

Treatment Modifications

- Mid-morning appointments
- Short (30–45 minutes) appointments
- Delay lengthy procedures until you evaluate patient's endurance
- Minimize stress
- Consider antianxiety medications
- If patient is in wheelchair
  - Determine if transfer is feasible

- Patient may need help staying upright in chair
  - Pillows, wedges
- Apraxia may make treatment difficult
  - Use mouth props
  - Gentle head hold
- Difficulty with swallowing/protecting airway/loss of gag reflex
  - Treat in upright/semisupine position
  - Rubber dam may be useful
  - Suction
- Pain control important
  - Obtain profound anesthesia
  - Limit use of vasoconstrictors especially with history of hypertension or use of nonselective beta blockers
    - Limit epinephrine to 0.04 mg (2 carpules of 1:100,000 or 4 carpules of 1:200,000 epinephrine) and levonordefrin to 0.2 mg
    - Avoid 1:50,000 concentrations of epinephrine in dental anesthetic and epinephrine-impregnated retraction cord.[27,48]

Restorative and Prosthetic Modifications

It may be difficult for the patient to tolerate being in the dental chair for the extended time that extensive restorative treatment takes. Treatment plans should be formulated taking into account the patient's ability to tolerate chair time, ability to maintain oral hygiene, aspiration risk, and need to replace missing teeth. Missing single teeth can be replaced using cantilevered resin-bonded bridges, which require little preparation of abutment teeth and may be easier for the patient to maintain than conventional fixed bridges.[49] Single-tooth implants can be considered as well. Removable prostheses must be carefully designed to accommodate loss of muscle control. Existing dentures can be relined or rebased if the patient's adaptive ability is in question. Partial dentures should be designed with ease of insertion and removal in mind. Notches can be placed on the labial flanges to aid in removal. Frameworks should be designed with the ability to add teeth easily. Addition of program of preventive maintenance must be in place before any complex restorative treatment is done.

- Try to conserve as much remaining dentition as possible
  - Periodontal splinting
- Evaluate whether missing teeth really need to be replaced
- Difficulty with daily placement and removal of removable prostheses
  - Fixed prostheses may be more desirable than removable
  - Avoid extensive bridgework unless oral hygiene is adequate
    - Hygienic pontics and cleansable embrasures
- Removable Prosthesis
  - Consider silicon-based removable if limited dexterity
  - Design to accommodate uneven occlusion
  - Maximum denture base extension to distribute forces more evenly
  - Zero degree teeth placed more buccally
  - Lateral and anteroposterior freedom on excursion
- Removable Partial Dentures
  - Make sure partial denture is easy to insert and remove
  - Paths of insertion and removal
  - Keep clasps simple and sturdy
    - Easily accessible

- ○ Finger grooves or removal devices
    - ■ To facilitate removal
- ○ Maintain guarded teeth as long as possible
    - ■ Design framework with ability to add teeth to framework
    - ■ When they fail, do not have to redo case

After stroke, patients may have difficulty maintaining good oral hygiene because of decreased dexterity and caregivers untrained in oral hygiene techniques. Secondary to swallowing impairment, patients may be on dietary supplements and thickened liquids that are not only high in sugar but have a consistency that causes them to stick to teeth. Loss of muscle tone and loss of sensation can cause food and debris to pool on the affected side, also increasing the amount of time that teeth are exposed to cariogenic foods, increasing the risk of tooth decay. Medication-induced xerostomia may also increase the rate of tooth decay, especially on root surfaces.

In addition to increased caries risk, the periodontal health of people with a history of a stroke is poorer than patients with no history of stroke. Patients tend to have higher levels of plaque, bleeding on probing, and attachment loss. There may be a correlation between stroke risk and periodontal disease, although definitive causation has not yet been proven.[50] It is possible that improved oral hygiene may reduce the incidence of stroke. The importance of good oral hygiene should be explained to both the patient and the patient's caregivers (if necessary) and individualized oral hygiene modifications made as needed. Preventive regimen should be aimed at reducing both the incidence of periodontal disease and caries and include regular recare visits as well as topical fluoride products.

- • Prevention Modifications
    - ○ Topical fluoride and remineralizing pastes[51]
    - ○ Fluoride varnish every recall
    - ○ Individualized preventive plans important
        - ■ Depends on residual physical deficit
    - ○ Patient may neglect affected side of mouth
    - ○ Go through homecare instructions carefully
    - ○ Give frequent specific feedback
- • Oral Hygiene Modifications
    - ○ Technical modifications for adequate oral hygiene
        - ■ Electric toothbrush, water irrigating devices, flossing aids
    - ○ Toothbrush modifications
    - ○ Enlarge toothbrush handle, modify on/off switch
    - ○ Floss threaders or interproximal brushes/cleaners
    - ○ Make sure oral hygiene tools are placed on "good side" of patient's sink
    - ○ Family and personal care providers need instruction

Patients can be managed in the dental office without complications as long as the patient is carefully monitored. Patients should be assessed for symptoms that could be barriers to maintaining good oral hygiene. Preventive strategies should take into account the patient's physical and cognitive deficits.

MULTIPLE SCLEROSIS
Description and Epidemiology

Multiple sclerosis (MS) is a chronic inflammatory disease of the central nervous system (CNS). It is characterized by recurrent episodes of neurologic dysfunction that are produced by demyelination of the axons located in the white matter of the CNS in multiple areas of the brain or spinal cord. It is one of the most common causes of nontraumatic disability among young and middle-aged adults. It can occur at any age, but most cases are diagnosed between the ages of 20 and 40.[52]

The number of people with MS in the United States is estimated to be approximately 400,000, with approximately 10,000 new cases diagnosed every year.[53] There appears to be increasing prevalence and incidence,[54] especially among women. MS is much more common in women than men, approximately 2 to 3 times more common in the relapsing-remitting form of MS (RRMS).[55] Although the exact etiology is unknown, MS is believed to be the result of complex interactions among genetic, infectious, and environmental factors[56] Decreased levels of vitamin D and sun exposure, smoking, Epstein-Barr virus, and human herpes virus 6 have all been hypothesized to play a role, as well as changes in the HLA-DRB1 gene.[57,58]

Clinical Presentation

MS is a progressive disease characterized with attacks or exacerbations that reflect CNS involvement. The symptoms may be insidious or acute and episodes occur months or years apart with different neurologic symptoms. Presenting symptoms include weakness and sensory loss in one or more extremities, gait and balance alterations, and visual changes[59] (**Box 7**). The course is unpredictable and depends on the frequency and severity of the attacks. Permanent neurologic impairment may develop with repeated relapses or disease progression resulting in significant disability. Oral and facial manifestation can include trigeminal neuralgia, trigeminal sensory neuropathy, facial palsy, temporomandibular pain, and dysphagia[59,60] (**Box 8**).

Box 7
Common signs and symptoms of MS

- Fatigue (75%)
- Paroxysmal pain
- Spasticity/dystonic spasms
- Vertigo
- Tremor
- Double vision/vision loss
- Weakness
- Dizziness/unsteadiness
- Numbness/tingling
- Ataxia
- Heat intolerance
- Memory change
- Cognitive dysfunction (attention span, concentration, memory)
- Depression
- Speech disturbance
- Bladder/bowel dysfunction

Box 8
Medications used in the treatment of MS

Disease-Modifying Drugs (DMD)

Aubagio (teriflunomide)

Avonex (interferon beta-1a)

Betaseron (interferon beta-1b)

Copaxone (glatiramer acetate)

Extavia (interferon beta-1b)

Gilenya (fingolimod)

Lemtrada (alemtuzumab)

Novantrone (mitoxantrone)

Plegridy (peginterferon beta-1a)

Rebif (interferon beta-1a)

Tecfidera (dimethyl fumarate)

Tysabri (natalizumab)

Acute exacerbations

3 to 5 days of intravenous high-dose corticosteroids

Spasticity

Dantrium (dantrolene)[a]

Klonopin (clonazepam)[a]

Lioresal (baclofen)[a]

Valium (diazepam)

Zanaflex (tizanidine)

Fatigue

Symmetrel (amantadine)[a]

Provigil (modafinil)

Prozac (fluoxetine)

Bladder control

Anticholinergics[a]

Botox

Walking difficulty

Ampyra (dalfampridine)

Pain

Elavil (amitriptyline)[a]

Klonopin (clonazepam)[a]

Neurontin (gabapentin)

Pamelor (nortriptyline)

Tegretol (carbamazepine)

Depression

Selective serotonin reuptake inhibitor[a]

Tricyclic antidepressant[a]

[a] May cause xerostomia.

Clinical course of the disease may vary, but generally there are 4 clinical types (**Fig. 1**):

RRMS
- 85% of all cases
- Women >> men
- Acute attacks of increased disease activity and worsening symptoms followed by remissions
- Symptoms may improve or disappear during remission

Secondary-progressive MS (SPMS)
- RRMS followed by a change in clinical course to progressive deterioration

Primary-progressive MS (PPMS)
- Approximately 10% of cases
- Women = men
- Steady progression of disease with no relapses or remissions
- Later onset (between the ages of 35 and 39)

Progressive-relapsing MS (PRMS)
- Approximately 5% of cases
- Clear relapses combined with a steady progression of the disease

Medical Management

Treatment and management of MS is aimed primarily at treating acute exacerbations, relieving symptoms of the disease, and preventing disease progression (**Box 9**). Acute attacks are generally managed with high doses of corticosteroids (both oral and intravenous) to provide symptomatic relief, shorten the duration of the attack, and accelerate recovery from the relapse. Disease-modifying drugs are used to reduce the frequency of relapses and reduce the progression of the disease by modulating the immune system. Other therapies are used to relieve or modify the symptoms of MS, such as spasticity, fatigue, bladder dysfunction, and paroxysmal pain.[62,63]

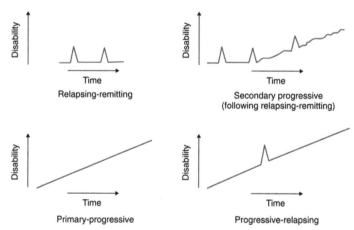

Fig. 1. Illustration of the most common different clinical courses of multiple sclerosis. (*From* Hersh CM, Fox RJ. Multiple sclerosis. Cleveland Clinic Center for Continuing Education. 2014. Available at: http://www.clevelandclinicmeded.com/medicalpubs/diseasemanagement/ neurology/multiple_sclerosis/; *Adapted from* Lublin FD, Reingold SC. Defining the clinical course of multiple sclerosis: results of an international survey. Neurology 1996;46:907–11.)

Box 9
Oral and facial manifestations of MS

- Sensory neuropathy
  - V2/V3
  - Sudden onset
- Progressive numbness of orofacial structures
  - Lower lip and chin
- Dysarthria
- Facial paralysis
- Bell palsy
- Trigeminal neuralgia (TN)
  - 400 times more likely in MS than general population[61]
  - May be presenting symptom of MS
  - Younger age than typical TN patient (<50 years old)
  - May be bilateral
  - Trigger zones may be absent

Dental Management

The optimal time to treat patients is during periods of remission. Only emergency care should be considered during acute exacerbations. There are no contraindications to dental care other than those related to any neurologic impairment present and potential side effects of medications used to treat MS. Patients with stable disease and limited motor impairment can receive routine dental care. Patients with more advanced symptoms may require changes in the position of the dental chair during treatment and help transferring to and from the dental chair. Altered manual dexterity and difficulty with oral hygiene maintenance may impact prosthetic and reconstructive treatment planning. Oral hygiene instructions and preventive regimens may need to be tailored for patients with physical deficits or those taking medications that cause xerostomia.

Treatment Considerations

- Dictated by level of motor impairment
- Patients undergoing acute relapse
  - No elective dental care
- Periods of remission
  - Optimum time to treat
- Medication considerations
  - Mood stabilizers, antispasmodics, amantadine, anticholinergics
    - Xerostomia
  - Corticosteroids/Immunosuppressant
    - Increased risk of infections

Treatment planning modifications

- Assess level of fatigue
  - Short AM appointments
  - After patient has taken medications
- May have poor airway protection and absent gag reflexes
  - May aspirate on secretions
  - Treat in semisupine position

- ○ Suction, especially posterior pharynx
- ○ Ask patient to swallow frequently
- May have trouble localizing pain
  - ○ Be absolutely clear as to origin of discomfort before performing restorations, endodontics, or extractions
- Stable disease and little motor spasticity or weakness
  - ○ Routine dental care
- More advanced disease
  - ○ Help transferring to and from dental chair
  - ○ Use mouth prop/tongue retractor
- Difficulty maintaining oral hygiene
  - ○ Modifications in oral hygiene products to accommodate altered manual dexterity
    - Altered toothbrush handles
    - Electric toothbrushes
    - Floss aids
  - ○ Preventive regimens
    - More frequent recalls
    - Antimicrobial rinses
    - Fluoride supplementation
- Care with reconstructive and complicated prosthetic procedures

PARKINSON DISEASE
Description and Epidemiology

In 1817 in his "Essay on the Shaking Palsy," James Parkinson described a condition that was characterized by rigidity and bradykinesia accompanied by a tremor at rest that came to be called Parkinson disease (PD). It is a progressive neurologic condition resulting from the slow loss of dopaminergic neurons in the substantia nigra region of the brain. It is believed to be the result of genetic and environmental factors. Seven to 10 million individuals are affected worldwide and that number is expected to double by 2030. It affects more than 1 million people in the United States, with approximately 60,000 people newly diagnosed each year. This number does not account for the thousands of cases that go undetected.[64] Incidence of PD increases with age, but an estimated 5% to 10% of people with PD are diagnosed before the age of 40 (young-onset PD). PD ranks among most common late-life neurodegenerative diseases (after AD) and affects approximately 1.5% to 2.0% of people aged 60 years and older.[65] Men are 1.5 times more likely to have PD than women.

Clinical Presentation

Diagnosis is based on clinical observation, as there is no definitive diagnostic test or laboratory finding. The acronym TRAP is used for the 4 primary PD motor symptoms (resting tremor, akinesia/bradykinesia, rigidity, and postural instability).[66] Diagnosis is considered when a patient has at least 2 of these. Motor symptoms tend to be worse on the side where the symptoms first appear. Nonmotor symptoms can include anxiety and depression, cognitive decline, and homeostatic instability (**Box 10**). Seventy-five percent of patients with PD develop some form of cognitive deficits over time, including memory and mood disturbances, sleep disruption, and other behavioral and psychiatric problems with 35% or more developing PD-related dementia in advanced disease. Cognitive deficits tend to be worse for patients with predominant symptoms of bradykinesia and rigidity.

Box 10
Signs and symptoms of Parkinson disease (PD)

Features that help diagnose PD

- Three or more of the primary motor symptoms
- Unilateral onset
- Persistent asymmetry affecting the side of onset most
- Progressive symptoms
- Positive response to levodopa

Clinical manifestations of PD.

Primary motor symptoms

- Bradykinesia
- Muscular rigidity
- Resting tremor
- Postural instability not caused by primary visual, vestibular, cerebellar, or proprioceptive dysfunction

Additional Motor Symptoms

- Masked face
- Dysphagia and sialorrhea
- Decreased blinking
- Stooped posture
- Hypokinetic dysarthria
- Reduced gesturing while speaking
- Decreased arm swing
- Shuffling gait with shortened stride length
- Festination ("Parkinson's gait")

Nonmotor Symptoms Seen in PD

- Fatigue
- Sensory disturbances
- Anosmia/ageusia
- Dysautonomia
  - Excessive sweating
  - Increased salivation
  - Orthostatic hypotension
  - Constipation
  - Urinary dysfunction
- Dysphagia
- Glossodynia
- Bruxism
- Cognitive decline/dementia
- Psychosis
- Anxiety
- Depression
- Impulse control disorders
- Sleep disturbances
- Sexual dysfunction

PARKINSON DISEASE SYMPTOMS

The Movement Disorder Society Unified Parkinson's Disease Rating Scale (MDS-UPDRS) is the most commonly used scale in following the clinical progression of the disease and can provide information on the disease severity and level of disability.[67] It includes evaluation of behavior and mood, monitored motor evaluation, evaluations of ADLs, complications of therapy and the Hoehn-Yahr staging of the severity of the disease (**Box 11**).[68]

Medical Management

There is no standard medical treatment for PD. Medical management is aimed at controlling symptoms and maintaining functional independence. Treatment protocols focus on increasing dopamine availability and preventing its breakdown by inhibiting acetylcholine by using neuroprotective therapies, dopamine agonists, levodopa/carbidopa levodopa alone, or with the addition of catechol-O-methyltransferase (COMT) inhibitors. Medications are also used to provide symptomatic relief (**Table 2**). Surgical intervention, such as deep brain stimulation and ablative thalamotomy, are generally reserved for advanced disease.[69,70]

Stretching, strengthening, and balance training may improve gait speed, balance, and participation in ADLs. Physical therapy, such as ballroom dancing and Tai Chi, appear to help patients maintain and regain balance, flexibility, and mobility.[71,72]

Dental Management

The progressive nature of PD should be considered when developing treatment options. Early and aggressive intervention to optimize patients' oral health and minimize potential complications should be done as early as possible in the PD process because of decreasing ability to cooperate later in the disease. Patients should be assessed for symptoms that could be barriers to maintaining good oral hygiene. Preventive strategies should take into account the patient's physical and cognitive deficits.

Treatment modifications

- Informed consent
  ○ Make sure patient is capable of giving consent
  ○ May need to obtain from caregiver if cognitive deficits present
- Treat in the morning
- Appointments 60 to 90 minutes after taking medications

Box 11
Hoehn and Yahr scale

I. Unilateral disease

II. Bilateral disease

III. Postural instability-mild

IV. Postural instability-marked

V. No independent ambulation

Data from Hoehn MM, Yahr MD. Parkinsonism: onset, progression, and mortality—1967. Neurology 1998;50(2):318–33.

Table 2
Treatment of Parkinson disease

Pharmacologic Management	Side Effects

Tremor control
  Amantadine (Symmetrel)
  Trihexyphenidyl (Artane)
  Benztropine (Cogentin)
  Propranolol (nonselective beta blocker)
	• Anticholinergic effects
	  ○ Dry mouth
	  ○ Drowsiness/sedation
	• Hypotension
	• Cognitive impairment

Dopamine precursor
  Levodopa/Carbidopa
  Sinemet,
  Parcopa,
  Stalevo,
  Rytary
	• Nausea, vomiting
	• Loss of appetite
	• Orthostatic hypotension
	• Dyskinesia
	• Bruxism
	• Confusion/delirium
	• Constipation
	• Dry mouth
	• Headache

Dopamine agonists
  Pramipexole (Mirapex)
  Ropinirole (Requip)
  Apomorphine (Apokyn)
  Rotigotine (Neupro)
	Side effects similar to levodopa

Monoamine oxidase-B inhibitor
  Prevent breakdown of dopamine
  Selegiline (Eldepryl)
  Rasagiline (Azilect)
  Zydis selegiline HCL (Zelapar)
	• Nausea
	• Dry mouth
	• Lightheadedness
	• Constipation
	• Agitation
	• Insomnia
	• Vivid dreams and hallucinations

Catechol-O-methyltransferase inhibitors
  Taken in combination with levodopa/
    carbidopa
  Entacapone (Comtan)
  Tolcapone (Tasmar)
	• Nausea and vomiting
	• Diarrhea
	• Enhanced side effects of levodopa,
	  especially dyskinesia
	• Orthostatic hypotension

Medication to improve cognitive changes
  Rivastigmine (Exelon)
  Donepezil (Aricept)
  Galantamine (Razadyne)
  Memantine (Namenda)
	• Nausea
	• Vomiting
	• Diarrhea

Nonpharmacologic Interventions

- Surgical intervention
  - Deep brain stimulation
  - Thalamotomy and pallidotomy
- Physical therapy
  - Yoga, bike riding, Tai chi, dancing

Data from Ahlskog JE. Parkinson's disease treatment guide for physicians. New York: Oxford University Press; 2009; and Goetz CG, Poewe W, Rascol O, et al. Evidence-based medical review update: pharmacological and surgical treatments of Parkinson's disease: 2001 to 2004. Mov Disord. 2005;20:523–39.

- Keep appointment short (<45 minutes)
  - Stress increases tremors/muscle rigidity
  - Break longer procedures into shorter pieces
  - May be difficult for patient to keep mouth open for extended periods

- ■ Mouth props or bite blocks, frequent breaks
- Poor airway protection
  - ○ Avoid reclining chair more than 45°
- Dysphagia and impaired cough/gag reflex
  - ○ Secretions and aspiration
  - ○ Use rubber dam
  - ○ Suction placed under dam to prevent saliva build-up
- Masklike face
  - ○ Difficulty knowing what patient is feeling
- Involuntary movements
  - ○ Mouth props
  - ○ Care with rotary instruments
  - ○ Soft arm and foot restraints
  - ○ Hand holding and head stabilization
  - ○ Sedation may be necessary
- Levodopa/COMT inhibitors/dopamine agonists
  - ○ Orthostatic hypotension
  - ○ Assist patient to and from chair
  - ○ Do not alter dental chair position too rapidly
- Bruxism (parkinsonian tremors/levodopa)
  - ○ Restorations with flat occlusion
  - ○ Metal occlusal surfaces
- Xerostomia-related cervical caries
  - ○ Glass ionomers and resin-modified glass ionomers
    - ■ Increased bonding to dentin and cementum
    - ■ Fluoride release
- Difficulty in control and retention of complete dentures
  - ○ Retain teeth even with guarded prognosis as long as possible
  - ○ Consider implant-supported overdentures[73,74]

Drug interactions

- COMT and monoamine oxidase B (MAO-B) inhibitors
  - ○ Exaggerated and prolonged pressor response to epinephrine
- COMT inhibitor
  - ○ Limit local anesthesia with epinephrine to 2 carpules
  - ○ Careful aspiration to avoid intravascular injection
  - ○ Monitor vital signs after administration of first carpule
- MAO-B inhibitor
  - ○ No epinephrine

Oral hygiene/prevention

- Assess patient's ability to perform oral hygiene
- More frequent dental recare appointments
  - ○ Fluoride varnishes at each visit
- Oral hygiene modifications
  - ○ Electric toothbrushes
  - ○ Modified toothbrush handles
  - ○ Floss aides, interproximal cleaners
- Chlorhexidine and alcohol-containing mouthrinses contraindicated
  - ○ Difficulty with swishing/expectorating

- Involvement of caregiver as needed
- Medication-related xerostomia
  - Topical fluorides
  - Salivary substitutes

SUMMARY

Patients with neurologic disease require individualized management considerations depending on the extent of impairment and impact on functional capacity. Oral involvement tends to be significant and affects the oral health status of the patient. Oral health care providers should be aware of the oral signs and symptoms as well as treatment modifications that are necessary to ensure that dental care is delivered in a safe and efficient manner.

REFERENCES

1. What is dementia? Alzheimer's Association Web site. Available at: http://www.alz.org/what-is-dementia.asp. Accessed October 20, 2015.
2. What is Alzheimers? Alzheimer's Association Web site. Available at: http://www.alz.org/alzheimers_disease_what_is_alzheimers.asp. Accessed October 20, 2015.
3. Hebert LE, Weuve J, Scherr PA, et al. Alzheimer disease in the United States (2010–2050) estimated using the 2010 census. Neurology 2013;80:1778–83.
4. 2015 Alzheimer's disease facts and figures. Alzheimer's Association website. Available at: http://www.alz.org/facts/. Accessed November 5, 2015.
5. Spires-Jones TL, Hyman BT. The intersection of amyloid beta and tau at synapses in Alzheimer's disease. Neuron 2014;82:756–71.
6. Eikelenboom P, Hoozemans JJ, Veerhuis R, et al. Whether, when and how chronic inflammation increases the risk of developing late-onset Alzheimer's disease. Alzheimers Res Ther 2012;4(3):15.
7. 10 early signs and symptoms of Alzheimer's. Alzheimer's Association Web site. Available at: www.alz.org/alzheimers_disease_10_signs_of_alzheimers.asp. Accessed October 24, 2015.
8. Reisberg B, Ferris SH, de Leon MJ, et al. The global deterioration scale for assessment of primary degenerative dementia. Am J Psychiatry 1982;139:1136–9.
9. Reisberg B, Ferris SH, de Leon MJ, et al. The stage specific temporal course of Alzheimer's disease: functional and behavioral concomitants based upon cross-sectional and longitudinal observation. Prog Clin Biol Res 1989;317:23–41.
10. Jack CR, Albert MS, Knopman DS, et al. Introduction to the recommendations from the National Institute on Aging–Alzheimer's Association workgroups on diagnostic guidelines for Alzheimer's disease. Alzheimers Dement 2011;7:257–62.
11. Turner LN, Balasubramaniam R, Hersh EV, et al. Drug therapy in Alzheimer disease: an update for the oral health care provider. Oral Surg Oral Med Oral Pathol Oral Radiol Endod 2008;106:467–76.
12. Balasubramaniam R, Ram S. Orofacial movement disorders. Oral Maxillofacial Surg Clin N Am 2008;20:273–85.
13. Wu B, Plassman BL, Crout RJ. Cognitive function and oral health among community-dwelling older adults. J Gerontol A Biol Sci Med Sci 2008;63A:495–500.
14. Kramer AR, Pirragliia E, Tsui W. Periodontal disease associates with higher brain amyloid load in normal elderly. Neurobiol Aging 2015;36:627–33.
15. Kramer AR, Craig RG, Dasanayake AP, et al. Inflammation and Alzheimer's disease: possible role of periodontal disease. Alzheimers Dement 2008;4:42–250.

16. Cicciu M, Matacena G, Signorino F, et al. Relationship between oral health and its impact on the quality life of Alzheimer's disease patients: a supportive care trial. Int J Clin Exp Med 2013;6:766–72.

17. Ribeiro GR, Costa JL, Ambrosano GM, et al. Oral health of the elderly with Alzheimer's disease. Oral Surg Oral Med Oral Pathol Oral Radiol 2012;114:338–43.

18. Ship JA, DeCarli C, Friedland RP, et al. Diminished submandibular salivary flow in dementia of the Alzheimer type. J Gerontol 1990;45(2):M61–5.

19. Friedlander AH, Norman DC, Mahler ME, et al. Alzheimer's disease: psychopathology, medical management and dental implications. J Am Dent Assoc 2006;137.9:1240–51.

20. Ettinger RL. Dental management of patients with Alzheimer's disease and other dementias. Gerodontology 2000;17.1:8–16.

21. Kocaelli H, Yaltirik M, Ozbas H, et al. Alzheimer's disease and dental management. Oral Surg Oral Med Oral Pathol Oral Radiol Endod 2002;93(5):521–4.

22. Mozaffarian D, Benjamin EJ, Go AS, et al. Heart disease and stroke statistics—2015 update: a report from the American Heart Association. Circulation 2015;131(4):e29–322.

23. CDC, NCHS. Underlying Cause of Death 1999-2013, released 2015. Data are from the Multiple Cause of Death Files, 1999-2013, as compiled from data provided by the 57 vital statistics jurisdictions through the Vital Statistics Cooperative Program. Available at: www.cdc.gov. Accessed October 25, 2015.

24. Centers for Disease Control and Prevention (CDC). Prevalence of stroke–United States, 2006-2010. MMWR Morb Mortal Wkly Rep 2012;61(20):379–82.

25. Seshadri S, Beiser A, Kelly-Hayes M, et al. The lifetime risk of stroke: estimates from the Framingham Study. Stroke 2006;37:345–50.

26. Ayala C, Croft JB, Greenlund KJ, et al. Sex differences in US mortality rates for stroke and stroke subtypes by race/ethnicity and age, 1995-1998. Stroke 2002;33:1197–201.

27. Fatahzadeh M, Glick M. Stroke: epidemiology, classification, risk factors, complications, diagnosis, prevention, and medical and dental management. Oral Surg Oral Med Oral Pathol Oral Radiol Endod 2006;102:180–91.

28. Little JW, Falace DA, Miller CS, et al. Neurologic disorders. In: Dental management of the medically compromised patient. 8th edition. St. Louis: Mosby; 2013. p. 494–521.

29. Grau AJ, Becher H, Ziegler CM, et al. Periodontal disease as a risk factor for ischemic stroke. Stroke 2004;35:496–501.

30. Zweifler RM. Management of acute stroke. South Med J 2003;96(4):380–5.

31. Stroke: signs and symptoms. Available at: http://www.cdc.gov/stroke/signs_symptoms.htm. Accessed November 5, 2015.

32. Lawes CM. Blood pressure and stroke: an overview of published reviews. Stroke 2004;35:776–85.

33. Bushnell C, McCullough LD, Awad IA, et al, American Heart Association Stroke Council, Council on Cardiovascular and Stroke Nursing, Council on Clinical Cardiology, Council on Epidemiology and Prevention, Council for High Blood Pressure Research. Guidelines for the prevention of stroke: a statement for healthcare professionals from the American Heart Association/American Stroke Association. Stroke 2014;45:1545–88.

34. Goldstein LB, Bushnell CD, Adams RJ, et al. Guidelines for the primary prevention of stroke: a guideline for healthcare professionals from the American Heart Association/American Stroke Association. Stroke 2011;42:517–84.

35. Saver JL. Time is brain–quantified. Stroke 2006;37(1):263–6.

36. Wardlaw JM, Murray V, Berge E, et al. Recombinant tissue plasminogen activator for acute ischaemic stroke: an updated systematic review and meta-analysis. Lancet 2012;379(9834):2364–72.
37. Marler JR, Lyden PD. The NINDS t-PA for acute stroke protocol. In: Lyden PD, editor. Thrombolytic therapy for stroke. Totowa (NJ): Humana; 2001. p. 297–308.
38. Jovin TG, Chamorro A, Cobo E, et al. Thrombectomy within 8 hours after symptom onset in ischemic stroke. N Engl J Med 2015;372:2296–306.
39. Badhiwala JH, Nassiri F, Alhazzani W, et al. Thrombectomy for acute ischemic stroke. JAMA 2015;314(17):1832–43.
40. Ciccone A, Valvassori L, Nichelatti M, et al. Endovascular treatment for acute ischemic stroke. N Engl J Med 2013;368(10):904–13.
41. Pendlebury ST, Mariz J, Bull L, et al. MoCA, ACE-R, and MMSE Versus the National Institute of Neurological Disorders and Stroke–Canadian Stroke Network Vascular Cognitive Impairment Harmonization Standards Neuropsychological Battery After TIA and Stroke. Stroke 2012;43(2):464–9.
42. Jokinen H, Melkas S, Ylikoski R, et al. Post-stroke cognitive impairment is common even after successful clinical recovery. Eur J Neurol 2015;22(9):1288–94.
43. Mupparapu M, Kim IH. Calcified carotid artery atheroma and stroke: a systematic review. J Am Dent Assoc 2007;138:483–92.
44. Minassian C, Kim IH. Invasive dental treatment and risk for vascular events: a self-controlled case series. Ann Intern Med 2010;153:499–506.
45. Elad S, Zadik Y, Kaufman E, et al. A new management approach for dental treatment after a cerebrovascular event: a comparative retrospective study. Oral Surg Oral Med Oral Pathol Oral Radiol Endod 2010;110:145–50.
46. Armstrong MJ, Gronseth G, Anderson DC, et al. Summary of evidence-based guideline: Periprocedural management of antithrombotic medications in patients with ischemic cerebrovascular disease: Report of the Guideline Development Subcommittee of the American Academy of Neurology. Neurology 2013;80:2065–9.
47. Singh SH. Dysphagia in stroke patients. Postgrad Med J 2006;82:383–91, 2065–9.
48. Napeñas JJ, Kujan O, Arduino PG, et al. World Workshop on Oral Medicine VI: controversies regarding dental management of medically complex patients: assessment of current recommendations. Oral Surg Oral Med Oral Pathol Oral Radiol 2015;120(2):207–26.
49. British Society of Gerodontology. Guidelines for the oral healthcare of stroke survivors. 2010. Available at: www.gerodontology.com/forms/stroke_guidelines.pdf. Accessed October 20, 2015.
50. Lockhart PB, Bolger AF, Papapanou PN, et al. Periodontal disease and atherosclerotic vascular disease: does the evidence support an independent association? A scientific statement from the American Heart Association. Circulation 2012;125(20):2520–44.
51. Hayes M. Topical agents for root caries prevention. Evid Based Dent 2015;16(1):10–1.
52. Noonan CW, Kathman SJ, White MC. Prevalence estimates for MS in the United States and evidence of an increasing trend for women. Neurology 2002;58:136–8.
53. MS statistics. Available at: http://multiplesclerosis.net/what-is-ms/statistics/. Accessed October 27, 2015.
54. Koch-Henriksen N, Sorensen PS. The changing demographic pattern of multiple sclerosis epidemiology. Lancet Neurol 2011;9:520–32.

55. Ontaneda D, Fox RJ, Chataway J. Clinical trials in progressive multiple sclerosis: lessons learned and future perspectives. Lancet Neurol 2015;14:208–22.

56. Mahad DH, Trapp BD, Lassmann H. Pathological mechanisms in progressive multiple sclerosis. Lancet Neurol 2015;14(2):183–93.

57. Cree BA. Multiple sclerosis genetics. Handb Clin Neurol 2014;122:193–209.

58. Belbasis L, Bellou V, Evangelou E, et al. Environmental risk factors and multiple sclerosis: an umbrella review of systematic reviews and meta-analyses. Lancet Neurol 2015;14(3):263–73.

59. Fischer DJ, Epstein JB, Klasser G. Multiple sclerosis: an update for oral health care providers. Oral Surg Oral Med Oral Pathol Oral Radiol Endod 2009; 108(3):318–27.

60. Chemaly D, Lefrançois A, Pérusse R. Oral and maxillofacial manifestations of multiple sclerosis. J Can Dent Assoc 2002;66:600–5.

61. Osterberg A, Voivie J, Thuomas KA. Central pain in multiple sclerosis—prevalence and clinical characteristics. Eur J Pain 2005;9:531–42.

62. Killestein J, Rudick RA, Polman CH. Oral treatment for multiple sclerosis. Lancet Neurol 2011;10(11):1026–34.

63. Michel L, Larochelle C, Prat A. Update on treatments in multiple sclerosis. Presse Med 2015;44(4 Pt 2):e137–51. Available at: http://dx.doi.org/10.1016/j.lpm.2015. 02.008. Accessed November 5, 2015.

64. Parkinson's disease. National Institute of Neurological Disorders and Stroke. Available at: http://www.ninds.nih.gov/disorders/parkinsons_disease/parkinsons_ disease.htm. Accessed October 27, 2015.

65. Nussbaum RL, Ellis CE. Alzheimer's disease and Parkinson's disease. N Engl J Med 2003;348:1356–64.

66. Alvarez MV, Evidente VG, Driver-Dunckley ED. Differentiating Parkinson's disease from other parkinsonian disorders. Semin Neurol 2007;27(4):356–62.

67. Miyasaki JM, Shannon K, Voon V, et al, Quality Standards Subcommittee of the American Academy of Neurology. Practice parameter: evaluation and treatment of depression, psychosis, and dementia in Parkinson disease (an evidence-based review): report of the Quality Standards Subcommittee of the American Academy of Neurology. Neurology 2006;66(7):996–1002.

68. Goetz CG, Tilley BC, Shaftman SR, et al. Movement Disorder Society-sponsored revision of the Unified Parkinson's Disease Rating Scale (MDS-UPDRS): scale presentation and clinimetric testing results. Mov Disord 2008;23:2129–70.

69. Olanow CW, Watts RL, Koller WC. An algorithm (decision tree) for the management of Parkinson's disease: treatment guidelines. Neurology 2001;56(Suppl 5): S1–88.

70. Koller WC, Pahwa R, Lyons KE, et al. Surgical treatment of Parkinson's disease [review]. J Neurol Sci 2009;167:1–10.

71. Deane KH, Jones D, Playford ED, et al. Physiotherapy for patients with Parkinson's disease: a comparison of techniques. Cochrane Database Syst Rev 2001;(3):CD002817.

72. Ahlskog JE. Does exercise have a neuroprotective effect in Parkinson disease? Neurology 2011;77(3):288–94.

73. Bakke M, Larsen SL, Lautrup C, et al. Orofacial function and oral health in patients with Parkinson's disease. Eur J Oral Sci 2011;119:27–32.

74. Packer M, Nikitin V, Coward T, et al. The potential benefits of dental implants on the oral health quality of life of people with Parkinson's disease. Gerodontology 2009;26:11–8.

The Special Needs of Preterm Children – An Oral Health Perspective

Annetta Kit Lam Tsang, BDSc (Hons), GCClinDent, GCEd(HE), MScMed(Pain Mgt), DClinDent (Paed Dent), PhD[a,b,*]

KEYWORDS

- Preterm • Low birthweight • Children • Dental • Oral health • Teeth • Malocclusion

KEY POINTS

- Preterm low birthweight children are at higher risks of orodental anomalies and acquired oral conditions.
- Oral health care for preterm children should commence as early as possible to enable early risk assessment, detection, and management of orodental anomalies and prevention of acquired oral conditions, through the establishment of a dental home.
- Parents and carers of preterm children need to be provided with timely advice and support regarding oral health in the context of general health, growth, and well-being; these are best achieved interprofessionally, with the help of non–dental health practitioners, to enable reinforcement.

INTRODUCTION

Preterm birth is defined by the World Health Organization as "a birth that occurs before 37 completed weeks of gestation or less than 259 days since the first day of the mothers' last menstrual period" (**Table 1**).[1] The current incidence is estimated to be 11% globally and the prevalence is increasing.[2–4] It has been estimated that approximately 15 million preterm births occur each year globally and, of these, more than 80% are classified as premature births and the rest as very premature or extremely premature births (see **Table 1**).[5] More male infants are born premature than female infants.[1,5,6] Male preterm infants have higher mortality and morbidity than female preterm infants.[5,6]

The morbidity and mortality rates of preterm births increase with decreasing gestational ages.[1] Infants born before or at 25 weeks are at highest risks of severe lifelong

[a] Gold Coast Oral Health Service, Gold Coast University Hospital, 1 Hospital Boulevard, Southport, Queensland 4215, Australia; [b] Griffith Health, Griffith University, Gold Coast Campus, Queensland 4222, Australia
* Gold Coast Oral Health Service, Gold Coast University Hospital, 1 Hospital Boulevard, Southport, Queensland 4215, Australia.
E-mail addresses: annetta.tsang@health.qld.gov.au; a.tsang@griffith.edu.au

Dent Clin N Am 60 (2016) 737–756
http://dx.doi.org/10.1016/j.cden.2016.02.005
0011-8532/16/$ – see front matter
dental.theclinics.com

Table 1
Classification of preterm infants according to gestational age and birthweight

Gestational Age	<28 wk	Extremely premature
	28 to <32 wk	Very premature
	32 to <37 wk	Premature
Birthweight	<2500 g	Low birthweight
	<1500 g	Very low birthweight
	<1000 g	Extremely low birthweight

Data from World Health Organization (WHO). International statistical classification of diseases and related health problems: instruction manual. Geneva (Switzerland): World Health Organization; 2004; and World Health Organization (WHO). Born too soon; the global action report on preterm birth. Geneva (Switzerland): World Health Organization; 2012.

impairment and have the lowest survival rates (**Fig. 1**).[1] In addition to gestational age, morbidity and mortality also increase with decreasing birthweights (see **Table 1**).[7] Most common causes for mortality among low birthweight and very-low-birthweight infants are prematurity and intrauterine growth restriction.[8] Infants born very or extremely premature with low birthweight, very low birthweight, or extremely low birthweight have higher mortality and morbidity risks than infants born small for gestational age at term.[5]

Short-term and-long term morbidities that occur among preterm infants vary enormously (**Box 1**). Frequently, morbidities are related to the immaturity of their organs and complications as a result of concurrent medical conditions and/or interventions.[8,9] Regardless of severity of prematurity or low birthweight, preterm infants are reported to have increased risk of short-term and long-term complications, including cerebral palsy, compromised neurodevelopmental outcomes, and chronic medical needs compared with their full-term counterparts (see **Box 1**).[5,7–14]

Effects of preterm birth on oral structures vary from infant to infant, depending on several factors, including gestational age, birthweight, postnatal medical complications and interventions, and growth and developmental complications (**Box 2**).[10,15,16] The risks of certain orodental manifestations are higher among preterm infants compared with full-term infants.[10,15,16]

COMMON ADVERSE EFFECTS ON THE ORODENTAL STRUCTURES AMONG PRETERM INFANTS
Developmental Enamel Defects

The prevalence of developmental enamel defects may be as high as 96% among infants born preterm and/or very low birthweight and extremely low birthweight.[15,17–21]

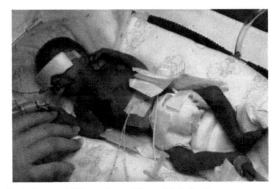

Fig. 1. Preterm infant, born at 25 weeks, with oral intubation.

Box 1
Common systemic morbidities of the preterm infant

Neurologic and neurodevelopmental

Cerebral palsy

Cognitive impairment

Epilepsy

Intraventricular hemorrhage

Cardiovascular and respiratory

Apnea

Bronchopulmonary dysplasia

Congestive cardiac failure

Patent ductus arteriosus

Respiratory distress syndrome

Gastrointestinal and endocrinological

Gastroesophageal reflux

Hyperbilirubinemia

Hypocalcemia

Hypoglycemia

Malabsorption

Necrotizing enterocolitis

Hematological and immunologic

Anemia

Infections

Sepsis

Sensory and other

Extrauterine growth restriction

Hearing impairment

Hypothermia

Motor deficits

Oral aversion

Retinopathy

Data from Refs.[7–14]

The incidence and severity of developmental enamel defects are highest among the sickest preterm infants and preterm infants with congenital conditions or syndromes.[15,22,23]

The most commonly affected teeth are the primary incisors, molars, and canines (**Figs. 2–4**).[19,24–26] Maxillary teeth tend to be more frequently affected than mandibular.[19,24,25] Developmental enamel defects of the permanent incisors and first molars are also reported to be more prevalent among preterm infants, especially if medications, such as amoxicillin, were used frequently in early life (**Figs. 5** and **6**).[10,27,28]

> **Box 2**
> **Common adverse effects on the orodental structures from prematurity**
>
> - Delayed eruption of primary teeth
> - Delayed development of permanent teeth
> - Dental arch distortions
> - Developmental enamel defects
> - Early colonization of cariogenic bacteria
> - Malocclusion
> - Palatal deformities
> - Tooth crown anomalies
> - Tooth number anomalies
> - Tooth size anomalies
>
> *Data from* Refs.[10,15,16]

Enamel defects are likely associated with local trauma and calcium homeostatic imbalance during the prenatal and postnatal periods, leading to disturbances during enamel matrix formation and mineralization.[29] Chemical analysis of primary teeth obtained from preterm infants indicated that the calcium:carbon ratio of the enamel surfaces was significantly lower (and therefore more porous) in preterm infants compared with full-term controls.[30] Light and scanning electron microscope analyses also concurred that the enamel of preterm infants is thinner than in full-term infants.[31] Even after a period of catch-up, postnatally formed enamel could not adequately compensate prenatal enamel.[31] Merheb and coworkers[32] added that the occurrence of enamel hypoplasia is significantly higher among very-low-birthweight infants with lower serum phosphorous levels. Due to the multifactorial nature of the risks and etiology of developmental enamel defects, these defects may present as subtle changes to enamel opacity due to disruptions in mineralization or maturation of the enamel matrix, as quantitative loss of enamel (ie, enamel hypoplasia), or, often, as a combination of both qualitative and quantitative changes.

Etiologic factors attributed to the development of enamel defects among preterm infants include disruption to amelogenesis and enamel matrix formation and

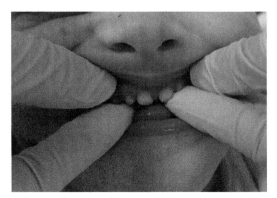

Fig. 2. Developmental enamel defect affecting the right maxillary primary central incisor.

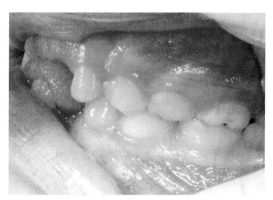

Fig. 3. Developmental enamel defects affecting the buccal surfaces of the maxillary and mandibular primary second molars in a child.

mineralization in utero and postnatally, especially in the presence of stress, intrauterine or extrauterine growth restriction, maternal systemic illnesses, and medications during pregnancy; infant systemic illnesses and medications postnatally; metabolic derangements during and beyond the neonatal period; and local trauma.[10,15,33–38] In the past, enamel defects among preterm infants were specifically attributed to localized trauma associated with laryngoscope, endotracheal intubation, and oral or nasogastric tube

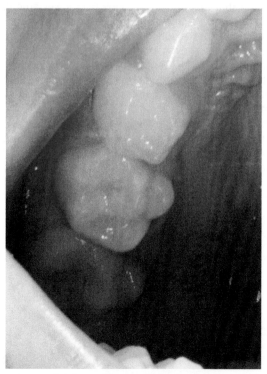

Fig. 4. Developmental enamel defects affecting the occlusal surface of the maxillary primary second molar.

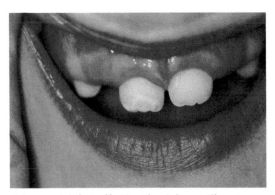

Fig. 5. Developmental enamel defect affecting the right maxillary permanent central incisor.

feeds.[10,15,22,33,35–39] Oral intubation, however, is now frequently replaced by nasal intubation, resulting in a reduced occurrence of enamel defects of this etiology.[10,16,20] Risks of enamel defects affecting both primary and permanent teeth are further increased by neonatal complications, malnutrition, orodental trauma, fevers, infections, medical conditions, and medications.[15,39]

Dental Caries

The occurrence of dental caries in the primary and permanent dentitions of preterm infants is generally regarded as similar to those born full term.[29,34,40–43] Gravina and coworkers[43] indicated that primary teeth caries was lower among preterm infants compared with full-term infants and suggested that this may be related to earlier and more regular access to oral examinations.

The risks of dental caries, however, in particular, early childhood caries (defined by the American Academy of Pediatric Dentistry [AAPD] as "the presence of one or more decayed [noncavitated or cavitated lesions], missing [due to caries], or filled tooth surfaces in any primary tooth in a child under the age of six"[44]) are potentially higher among preterm infants (**Fig. 7**).

The potential increased caries risk among preterm infants may be due to factors that modify the oral flora and demineralization versus remineralization equilibrium, such as medical conditions and medications, immature or impaired immunity, fetal growth retardation, enamel defects, feeding and dietary factors, and cognitive and behavioral factors.[3,19,20,34,45]

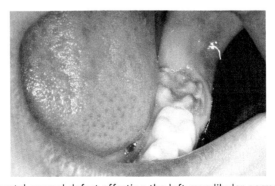

Fig. 6. Developmental enamel defect affecting the left mandibular permanent first molar.

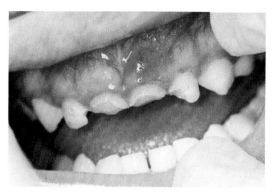

Fig. 7. Maxillary primary anterior teeth affected by HAS-ECC.

For example, immature immunity may increase the ease of early colonization of cariogenic bacteria, such as mutans streptococci.[46] Enamel defects may increase the ease of early colonization of cariogenic bacteria due to roughened tooth surfaces as well as increase the ease of structural breakdown due to reduced enamel quantity and quality.[19,47,48] Preterm infants are more likely to require medications for a prolonged period of time and these medications may be acidic and/or contain a high percentage of sucrose, thereby promoting the establishment of a more acidogenic and cariogenic oral flora.[49–51] Transmission-related behaviors, such as increased maternal contact during feeding, may also lead to greater likelihood of earlier colonization of cariogenic bacteria among predentate preterm infants.[46,52] In addition, weight gain is often more of a concern for preterm infants than for their full-term counterparts, resulting in greater likelihood of on-demand feeding, frequent feeding, and night feeding and the consumption of high-caloric infant formulae that are often higher in sugar content.[28,53] Preterm infants may be at risk of developing oral aversion due to various reasons, for example, prolonged nasogastric feeding, and this may enhance feeding, eating, and weaning difficulties as well as oral hygiene challenges.[45,53] Modified diets and feeding practices further increase risks of dental caries among preterm infants, especially in the presence of developmental enamel defects.[54] Mouth breathing, which occurs commonly among preterm infants with respiratory complications, has also been suggested to increase caries risk due to drying of the mouth, saliva evaporation, more adherent dental plaque, and reduced oral cleansing.[8,55,56]

Tooth Wear

Tooth wear (erosion, abrasion, and attrition) affecting the primary dentition is common.[57–59] Preterm infants have not been reported at higher risk of tooth wear compared with full-term infants. Preterm infants are at risk, however, of gastroesophageal reflux or vomiting and this, in turn, poses an increased risk to tooth wear.[8,59,60] Preterm infants who are exposed to extrinsic acids as a result of medications, frequent consumption of fresh and dried fruits and juice, and so forth are also at greater risks of erosion, especially in the presence of developmental enamel defects.[49,50,58,60] Enamel weakened by erosion may be at greater risk of attrition and abrasion as well as dental caries (**Fig. 8**).[57] In addition, preterm infants with neurosensory disorders, who are prone to parafunctional habits such as bruxism, may be at higher risk of attrition and abrasion.[50]

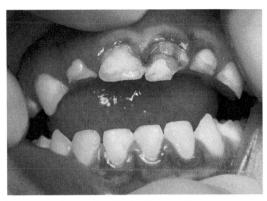

Fig. 8. Maxillary primary anterior teeth affected by developmental enamel defects, erosion, attrition, dental caries, and trauma.

Tooth Crown Anomalies

Primary tooth crown dimensions are reduced in preterm infants by approximately 10%.[61] The lower the birthweight, the smaller the tooth crown dimensions.[61,62] The change in primary tooth crown dimensions is likely associated with reduction in enamel in the presence of developmental enamel defects or mineral loss as a result of metabolic derangements, nutritional disturbances, and infections.[31,63] The same changes in tooth crown dimensions are not noted in the permanent dentition, which may be related to lessened physiologic disturbances in preterm infants as they catch up in growth postnatally.[39]

Developmental anomalies relating to tooth morphology (eg, dilaceration of crowns and roots of primary teeth and arrested tooth development) are associated with localized trauma to the underlying tooth germ/s as a result of significant pressure on the alveolar ridge during prolonged intubation and/or from laryngoscope (**Figs. 9** and **10**).[10,20,28,39]

Developmental anomalies relating to tooth number (eg, hypodontia and supernumerary) have also been reported to occur at greater frequency among preterm infants (see **Fig. 9**).[21] The risks of tooth number anomalies increase substantially among preterm infants born with a syndrome or cleft lip and/or cleft palate.[21]

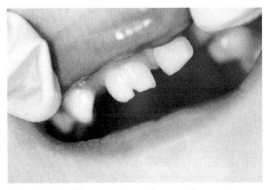

Fig. 9. Tooth crown anomaly affecting the right maxillary primary central incisor and congenitally missing primary lateral incisors.

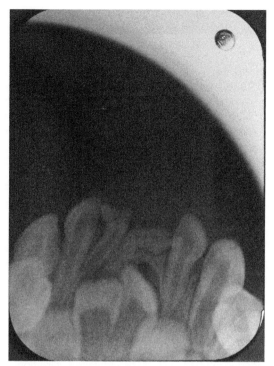

Fig. 10. Periapical radiograph showing tooth crown anomaly and noneruption of the left mandibular primary central incisor.

The risk of tooth crown discolorations may increase among preterm infants as a result of localized trauma and/or frequent or prolonged use of medications (eg, ciprofloxacin).[64] Extrinsic staining may also be more common among preterm infants as a result of certain medications or supplements (eg, liquid iron supplements) (**Fig. 11**).[8]

Eruption Delays

Delayed eruption of primary teeth is observed among preterm infants but catch-up later in infancy generally leads to eruption of permanent teeth at similar ages to those born full term. Delayed eruption of primary teeth is significantly associated with low

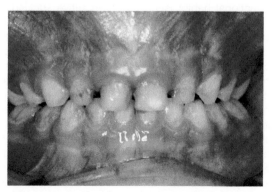

Fig. 11. Extrinsic staining associated with regular oral intake of liquid iron supplement.

birthweight, in particular birthweight less than 1000 g, and gestatational age less than 30 weeks.[65–67]

Palatal Deformities

Palatal deformities occur more commonly in preterm infants compared with their full-term counterparts.[68] Severe deformities, such as clefts, are usually detected antenatally during ultrasound screening. Postpartum, inspection of the oral cavity for anomalies, such as natal teeth, mucosal lesions, clefts of soft and hard palate, and bifid uvula, forms part of the newborn examination conducted by neonatologists and pediatricians.[8]

Palatal distortion, deepening, grooving, asymmetry, and narrowing are associated with significant external forces from prolonged endotracheal intubation and orogastric feeds.[10,22,39,69,70] Mild palatal distortion associated with intubation is usually transient, with deformities repaired through normal growth and remodeling.[10] Prolonged palatal deformities may contribute to malocclusion and/or malalignment and the need for early orthodontic assessment and treatment planning.[15,20,39,70,71]

Palatal deformities have also been attributed to persistent and prolonged non-nutritive sucking.[71,72] Non-nutritive sucking is used to reduce stress and promote weight gain and gastrointerestinal maturation and growth and, therefore, is often recommended to preterm infants.[8,73,74]

Dental Arch Distortions

Dental arch distortions, such as notching of the alveolar ridge, are reported more frequently among preterm infants compared with full-term infants. Dental arch distortions are primarily attributed to local pressure from intubation procedures and equipment as well as prolonged intubation.[16,70] The increased utilization of nasal intubation instead of oral intubation may reduce adverse effects on the oral cavity.[10,20,22,39]

Malocclusions

The prevalence of malocclusion is not thought significantly higher among children born preterm versus full term per se.[56] In contrast, Rythen and coworkers[16] noted, in their study of extremely preterm infants, a significantly higher frequency of Angle class II malocclusion and attributed this to dentoalveolar effects and medical conditions. Palatal and dentoalveolar deformities and tooth crown anomalies are associated with increased risks of malocclusion and these are common among preterm infants.[39,70,75] The changes of the palate and dentoaveolar complex, however, as a result of intubation have been reported to be transient and, by prepubertal stage, remodeling often has occurred and deformities resolved.[56,65]

Persistent parafunctional habits, such as non-nutritive sucking, including digits, thumbs, and pacifiers, further contribute to altered dentoskeletal development and malocclusion, such as narrowing of the palate, narrowing of the maxillary arch, posterior cross bites, open bites, proclination of the maxillary incisors, and retroclination of the mandibular incisors.[72,76–80] These developmental disturbances may pose a risk for preterm infants where non-nutritive sucking is encouraged to promote feeding and for its pacifying effects.[8,73,74] Once commenced, non-nutritive sucking habits tend to persist and if such habits extend past age 4 years, alternated dentoskeletal development and increased risk of malocclusion become significant.[79,80] On the other hand, spontaneous resolution of the altered dentoskeletal structures occurs if habit cessation occurs before age 6 years.[71,79,80] In addition, prolonged sucking beyond 6 hours per day poses the greatest malocclusion risks.[71]

Mouth breathing may also increase the risk of malocclusion, including mandibular retrusion, increased anterior facial height, cross bites, and anterior open bites.[79,80]

The frequency of inadequate nose breathing is high among preterm infants, especially in the presence of common medical conditions (eg, respiratory distress syndrome).[8,55,56]

Mode of feeding may also contribute to malocclusion.[56] Studies have reported lower incidences of anterior open bite and posterior cross bite among breastfeeding infants compared with bottle-feeding infants and attributed this to different patterns of muscle activity.[81–83]

PREVENTION AND MANAGEMENT STRATEGIES
Dental Home and Risk Assessment

Given that preterm infants, in particular, preterm infants with low birthweights, are at higher risks of oral conditions compared with infants born full-term and/or with normal birthweights, early dental consultation with a specialist pediatric dentist or general dentist experienced with managing young children may be of benefit. This is likely most beneficial when the pediatric dentist or general dentist contributes as part of a multidisciplinary growth and development health care team, so that anticipatory guidance, treatment planning, and prevention can be considered in the context of oral health as part of general health. Pediatricians, general medical practitioners, and community child health clinics can also contribute significantly to early risk assessment and increasing awareness of the importance of oral health in the context of general health, especially for medically compromised infants (**Table 2**).[42,50]

Table 2
Risk factors for common oral conditions affecting preterm infants

Oral Disease	Risk Factor Suggesting High Risk of Disease
Enamel defects	Very and extremely preterm infants Low, very low, and extremely low birthweights Chronic medical conditions Frequent or prolonged infections or high fevers Prolonged neonatal oral intubation needs
Dental caries	Poor parental oral health Presence of enamel defects Prolonged use of low pH and/or sugar-containing medications Visible plaque on teeth Infrequent/ineffective tooth brushing Fluoridated toothpaste not used On-demand/prolonged/night feeding (breast or formula) Grazing or continuous eating/drinking/snacking pattern
Tooth wear (erosion, attrition)	Presence of enamel defects Gastroesophageal reflux Frequent vomiting Neurosensory/neurodevelopmental disorders Reduced quantity and/or quality of saliva Excessive bruxism/grinding Prolonged use of low pH/acid-containing medications Prolonged use of xerostomia-inducing medications High exposure to dietary acids (foods and fluids)
Tooth, dental arch, palatal anomalies	Syndromes and complex medical conditions Prolonged neonatal oral intubation needs Prolonged non-nutritive sucking habits

Data from Refs.[15,16,20,29,39,42,44,52,54,58,60,61,79,80,84–87]

Even for healthy infants, the AAPD recommends establishment of a "dental home" for children "as early as six months of age, six months after the first tooth erupts and no later than 12 months of age" to enable timely risk assessment, anticipatory guidance, and customized prevention.[85,88]

Risk assessment of oral conditions should occur as early as possible and be reassessed continuously (see **Table 2**). Most oral conditions are multifactorial in etiology, with a large number of risk factors, and susceptible to change over time. A risk assessment pro forma, such as the AAPD caries-risk assessment forms[44,84] or the Caries Management by Risk Assessment forms,[89,90] may assist with the comparing risk changes from 1 time point to another. Once risks are identified, risk-based patient-centered at-home and in-office preventive strategies can be planned and implemented to optimize efficacy and cost-effectiveness.[44,84,85]

Anticipatory Guidance

Anticipatory guidance is providing relevant and timely information to parents and carers about their infant's approaching developmental stage, to increase awareness and understanding and promote self-efficacy (**Table 3**).[8] The American Academy of Pediatrics and AAPD recommend that ideally anticipatory guidance, covering general health, oral health, and wellness, should commence soon after pregnancy and be continued through infants' growth and developmental stages.[85] Anticipatory guidance may include providing information relating to type of social and community support available, resources for maternal health, and information for infant nurturing, such as milestones, feeding, sleeping, settling, hygiene, immunization, and safety.[8]

DEVELOPMENTAL ENAMEL DEFECTS

The presence of developmental enamel defects increases the likelihood of dentine exposure and hypersensitivity, dental caries, tooth wear, and, if anteriorly located, aesthetic concerns.[10,15,38,39,54,98] The presence of developmental enamel defects in the primary dentition exponentially increases the likelihood of early childhood caries, more specifically "hypoplasia-associated early childhood caries (HAS-ECC)" (see **Fig. 7**).[39,54,99] In addition, given that enamel formation of the permanent first molars and incisors occurs at similar times to that of second primary molars, the presence of enamel defects on the primary molars should indicate the need for more frequent follow-up because the risk of molar-incisor hypoplasia in the permanent dentition is increased.[39]

Early detection of enamel defects is critical to reducing hypersensitivity associated with loss of enamel and exposure of dentine as well as aesthetic compromises and allowing timely advice; intervention, such as surface sealants; and intensive fluoride therapy to prevent the onset and progression of dental caries and tooth wear. Dental examination of children at the age of 4 years may not be early enough to prevent breakdown of teeth affected by enamel defects, especially in the presence of dental caries and/or erosion.[99]

If enamel defects are evident, persistent use of Tooth Mousse (10% casein phosphopeptide–amorphous calcium phosphate [CPP-ACP]) has been recommended as an adjunct to fluoride, to aid with surface remineralization and build resistance against demineralization.[100–102] In cases of enamel defects including hypoplasia (ie, a quantitative loss of enamel), early protection with fissure and surface sealants or resin infiltration may be worthwhile.[103] Most importantly, parents and carers need to be educated about developmental enamel defects and the increased risks to oral diseases and methods of early prevention.

Table 3	
Suggested topics for age-appropriate oral health anticipatory guidance for preterm infants	
Antenatal	Family oral health
	Maternal oral health and preterm risks
	Oral bacteria and colonization
	Oral health and general health
	Common oral diseases: dental caries,
	tooth wear, periodontal disease
0–4 mo	Oral cleansing
	Different sugar content in different formula
	Use of pacifier
	Medications and oral health
4–6 mo	Teething
	Weaning
	Issues with juice
	Oral health friendly solids and fluids
	Avoidance of bottle in bed
6–12 mo	Oral health risk assessments
	Tooth eruption
	Tooth brushing
	Fluoride toothpaste
	Minimize grazing pattern of eating/drinking
	Cessation of on demand/prolonged/night feeding
	(breast or formula or fluids other than water)
1–2 y	Dental home
	Food choices in kindergarten/childcare and home
	Supplements (eg, iron and vitamins) and oral health
	Night-time routine and tooth brushing
	Drinking from an open cup or with a straw
	Reinforcing regular meal times and limiting snacking
	Fluoride varnish
	First aids for dental injuries
2–3 y	Healthy diets and good eating patterns
	Flossing/interdental cleaning
	Building dental confidence
	Preparing for pacifier cessation

Data from Refs.[8,53,85,91–97]

DENTAL CARIES

Given that preterm infants are potentially at greater risk of early childhood caries than their full-term counterparts due to multiple factors, including higher risk of enamel defects; medication-related issues, such as sugar content in medications and medication-induced xerostomia; high-caloric diets that are often also high in sugar, and so forth, caries risk assessment, early risk-based prevention, and anticipatory guidance are of high priority.

Preterm infants assessed as at high caries risk may benefit from preventive interventions, such as periodic professional application of fluoride varnish, in addition to twice-daily at home tooth brushing with a fluoridated children's toothpaste, a low refined-carbohydrate diet, and regular dental home visits.[96,97] In contrast, there seems to be a lack of evidence to support the use of remineralizing or antibacterial agents, such as xylitol, chlorhexidine, CPP-ACP, or sealants for the prevention of early childhood caries.[96]

Treatment is often indicated once cavitations are identified. Treatment options are essentially the same for all infants, preterm or otherwise. For preterm infants, however, additional factors, such as presence of enamel defects, frequent reflux or vomiting, and medication use, need to be considered. Comprehensive treatment of early childhood caries generally necessitates general anesthesia.[96] Restorations are preferred to extractions due to adverse effects, such as midline shifts, space issues, and aesthetic concerns with premature extraction of primary teeth.[71,104] For longevity and reduced likelihood of retreatment needs, extracoronal restorations, such as stainless steel crowns, composite resin crowns, and zirconia crowns, are recommended (**Fig. 12**).[105–107] Dental treatment under general anesthesia, however, does not alleviate future caries development; therefore, post-treatment follow-up of these high-risk preterm infants must be intensive and sustained.[96,97]

TOOTH WEAR

Tooth wear in primary teeth resulting in dentine exposure and symptoms increases with age; therefore, identification of risks and then implementing risk-based prevention is of utmost importance.[58,60,108] Agents, such as CPP-ACP and combined polyvalent metal ions with fluorides, have been suggested for the prevention of tooth wear, in particular erosion, through remineralization of surface enamel.[57,101,109,110] Severe tooth wear may render restoration, stainless steel crown, pulp therapy, or extraction necessary.[58,60]

TOOTH, DENTAL ARCH, PALATAL ANOMALIES, AND MALOCCLUSION

Preterm infants may be at greater risk of tooth anomalies, dental arch deformations, palatal anomalies, and malocclusion due to both systemic (eg, clefts and hypotonia) and local (eg, prolonged oral intubation and prolonged non-nutritive sucking habits) factors. Therefore, parents and carers should be advised of these possibilities to reduce anxiety and increase coping.

Prevention may or may not be possible, depending on risk factors. Interception and/or treatment options are available, however, and should be discussed with parents and carers where indicated. For example, orthodontic appliances are available to aid with cessation of non-nutritive sucking habits and interceptive orthodontics may be useful for expansion of the maxillary arch.[71,79,80]

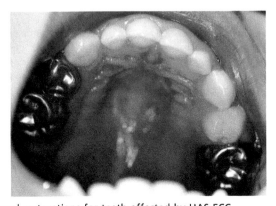

Fig. 12. Extracoronal restorations for teeth affected by HAS-ECC.

SUMMARY

Preterm infants, especially preterm infants with low, very low, or extremely low birth-weights, are at potentially higher risks of developmental oral anomalies and acquired oral conditions. These are not limited to the primary dentition but also may involve the permanent dentition. Furthermore, complications are not limited to teeth but also may affect anatomic structures, such as the palate. Strategies for optimizing the oral health of preterm infants should involve early risk assessment, risk-based patient-centered prevention, and early intervention. Management strategies that place oral health in the context of general health, involving primary carers and nondental health practitioners, should be considered for optimizing long-term outcomes.

REFERENCES

1. World Health Organization (WHO). International statistical classification of diseases and related health problems: instruction manual. Geneva (Switzerland): World Health Organization; 2004.
2. World Health Organization (WHO). Born too soon; the global action report on preterm birth. Geneva (Switzerland): World Health Organization; 2012.
3. Casey PH. Growth of low birthweight preterm children. Semin Perinatol 2008; 32(1):20–7.
4. Ong KK, Kenedy K, Castaneda Gutierrez E, et al. Postntal growth in preterm infants and later health outcomes: a systemic review. Acta Paediatr 2015;104(10): 974–86 [systematic review].
5. Blencowe H, Cousens S, Oestergaard MZ, et al. National, regional and worldwide estimates of preterm birth rates in the year 2010 with time trends since 1990 for selected countries: a systematic analysis and implications. Lancet 2012;379(9832):2162 [systematic review].
6. Kent AL, Wright IM, Abdel-Latif ME, et al. Mortality and adverse neurologic outcomes are greater in preterm male infants. Pediatrics 2012;129(1): 124–31.
7. Platt MJ. Outcomes in preterm infants. Public Health 2014;128(5):399–403.
8. Marcdante KJ, Kliegman RM, Jenson HB, et al. Nelson Essentials of pediatrics. 6th edition. Philadelphia: Saunders Elsevier; 2011. p. 28–30, 211–62.
9. Symington A, Pinelli J. Developmental care for promoting development and preventing morbidity in preterm infants. Cochrane Database Syst Rev 2006;(2):CD001814. [systematic review].
10. Seow WK. Effects of preterm birth on oral growth and development. Aust Dent J 1997;42(2):85–91.
11. O'Shea M. Cerebral palsy. Semin Perinatol 2008;32(1):35–41.
12. Dodrill P. Feeding difficulties in preterm infants. Infant Child Adolesc Nutr 2011; 3(6):324–31.
13. Teune MJ, Bakhuizen S, Bannerman CG, et al. A systematic review of severe morbidity in infants born late preterm. Am J Obstet Gynecol 2011;205(4): 374.e1–9 [systematic review].
14. Adams-Chapman I. Long-term impact of infection on the preterm neonate. Semin Perinatol 2012;36:462–70.
15. Nelson S, Albert JM, Geng C, et al. Increased enamel hypoplasia and very low birthweight infants. J Dent Res 2013;72:788–94.
16. Rythen M, Thilander B, Robertson A. Dento-alveolar characteristics in adolescents born extremely preterm. Eur J Orthod 2013;35:475–82.

17. Seow WK, Humphrys C, Tudehope DI. Increased prevalence of developmental dental defects in low-birth-weight children. A controlled study. Pediatr Dent 1987;9:221–5.
18. Fearne JM, Bryan EM, Ellman AM, et al. Enamel defects in the primary dentition of children born weighing less than 2000g. Braz Dent J 1990;168:433–7.
19. Lai PY, Seow WK, Tudehope DI, et al. Enamel hypoplasia and dental caries in very low birthweight children: a case controlled study. Pediatr Dent 1997;19:42–9.
20. Jacobsen PE, Haubeek D, Henriksen TB, et al. Developmental enamel defects in children born preterm: a systematic review. Eur J Oral Sci 2014;122:7–14 [systematic review].
21. Prokocimer T, Amir E, Blumer S, et al. Birth-weight, pregnancy term, pre-natal and natal complications related to child's dental anomalies. J Clin Pediatr Dent 2015;39(4):371–6.
22. Kopra DE, Davis EL. Prevalence of oral defect among neonatally intubated 3- to 5- and 7- to 10-year old children. Pediatr Dent 1991;113:349–55.
23. Wright JT, Carrion IA, Morris C. The molecular basis of hereditary enamel defects in humans. J Dent Res 2015;94(1):52–61.
24. Aine L, Backstrom MC, Maki R, et al. Enamel defects in primary and permanent teeth of children born prematurely. J Oral Pathol Med 2000;29:403–9.
25. Franco KM, Line SR, de Moura-Ribeiro MV. Prenatal and neonatal variables associated with enamel hypoplasia in deciduous teeth in low birthweight preterm infants. J Appl Oral Sci 2007;15(6):518–23.
26. Rythen M, Noren JG, Sabel N, et al. Morphological aspects of dental hard tissues in primary teeth from preterm infants. Int J Paediatr Dent 2008;18:397–406.
27. Hong L, Levy SM, Warren JJ, et al. Association between enamel hypoplasia and dental caries in primary secondary molars: a cohort study. Caries Res 2009;43(5):345–53.
28. Ferrini FR, Marba ST, Gaviao MB. Oral conditions in very low and extremely low birthweight children. J Dent Child (Chic) 2008;75:403–9.
29. Nelson S, Albert JM, Lombardi G, et al. Dental caries and enamel defects in very low birthweight adolescents. Caries Res 2010;44:509–18.
30. Rythen M, Sabel N, Dietz W, et al. Chemical aspects on dental hard tissues in primary teeth from preterm infants. Eur J Oral Sci 2010;118:389–95.
31. Seow WK, Young WG, Tsang AKL, et al. A study of primary dental enamel from preterm and fullterm children using light and scanning electron microscopy. Pediatr Dent 2005;27:374–9.
32. Merheb R, Arumugam C, Lee W, et al. Neonatal serum phosphorus levels and enamel defects in very-low-birth-weight infants. JPEN J Parenter Enteral Nutr 2015 [pii:0148607115573999]. [Epub ahead of print].
33. Noren JG, Ranggard L, Klienberg G, et al. Intubation and mineralisation disturbances in the enamel of primary teeth. Acta Odontol Scand 1993;51:271–5.
34. Shulman JD. Is there an association between low birthweight and caries in the primary dentition? Caries Res 2005;39:161–7.
35. Takaoka LA, Goulart AL, Kopelman BI, et al. Enamel defects in the complete primary dentition of children born at term and preterm. Pediatr Dent 2011;33(2):171–6.
36. Alves PV, Luiz RR. The influence of orotracheal intubation on the oral tissue development in preterm infants. Oral Health Prev Dent 2012;10(2):141–7.

37. Pinho JR, Filho FL, THomaz EB, et al. Are low birthweight, intrauterine growth restriction and preterm birth associated with enamel developmental defects? Pediatr Dent 2012;34:244–8.

38. Correa-Faria P, Martins-Junior PA, Viieira-Andrade RG, et al. Developmental defects of enamel in primary teeth: prevalence and associated factors. Int J Paediatr Dent 2013;23:173–9.

39. Salanitri S, Seow WK. Developmental enamel defects in the primary dentition: etiology and clinical management. Aust Dent J 2013;58:133–40.

40. Burt BA, Pai S. Does low birthweight increase the risk of caries? A systematic review. J Dent Educ 2001;65(10):1024–7 [systematic review].

41. Brogardh-Roth S, Stjernqvist K, Matsson L. Dental behavioral management problems and dental caries prevalence in 3- to 6-year-old Swedish children born preterm. Int J Paediatr Dent 2008;18:341–7.

42. Fontana M. The clinical, environmental and behavioral factors that foster early childhood caries: evidence for caries risk assessment. Pediatr Dent 2015; 37(3):217–25 [systematic review].

43. Gravina DB, Cruvinel VR, Azevedo TD, et al. Prevalence of dental caries in chidren born prematurely or at full term. Braz Oral Res 2006;20(4):353–7.

44. American Academy of Pediatric Dentistry. Policy on early childhood caries (ECC) – classifications, consequences and preventive strategies. 2014. Reference Manual v36; no.6. 2014/2015. 50–12. Available at: www.aapd.org/media/Policies_Guidelines/P_ECCClassifications.pdf. Accessed September 02, 2015.

45. Brogardh-Roth S, Stjernqvist K, Matsson L, et al. Parental perspectives on preterm children's oral health behavior and experience of dental care during preschool and early school years. Int J Paediatr Dent 2009;19:243–50.

46. Wan AK, Seow WK, Purdie DM, et al. Oral colonization of Streptococcus mutans in six-month-old predentate infants. J Dent Res 2001;80(12):2060–5.

47. Oliveira AFB, Chaves AMB, Rosenblatt A. The influence of enamel defects on the development of early childhood caries in a population with low socioeconomic status: a longitudinal study. Caries Res 2006;40(4):296–302.

48. Hong L, Levy SM, Warren JJ, et al. Association of amoxicillin use during early childhood with developmental tooth enamel defects. Arch Pediatr Adolesc Med 2005;159(10):943–8.

49. Bigeard L. The role of medication and sugars in pediatric dental patients. Dent Clin North Am 2000;44(3):443–56.

50. Foster H, Fitzgerald J. Dental disease in children with chronic illness. Arch Dis Child 2005;90:703–8.

51. Nankar M, Walimbe H, Ahmed bijle MN, et al. Comparative evaluation of cariogenic and erosive potential of commonly prescribed pediatric liquid medicaments: an in vitro study. J Contemp Dent Pract 2014;15(1):20–5.

52. Fontana M, Jackson R, Eckert G, et al. Identification of caries risk factors in toddlers. J Dent Res 2011;90:209–14.

53. Davenport ES, Litenas C, Barbayiannis P, et al. The effects of diet, breast-feeding and weaning on caries risk for pre-term and low birthweight children. Int J Paediatr Dent 2004;14:251–9.

54. Caufield PW, Li Y, Bromage TG. Hypoplasia-associated severe early childhood caries – a proposed definition. J Dent Res 2012;91(6):544–50.

55. Nascimento Filho E, Mayer M, Pontes P, et al. Caries prevalence, levels of mutans streptococci and gingival and plaque indices in 3.0- to 5.0-year-old mouth breathing children. Caries Res 2004;38:572–5.

56. Primozic J, Farcnik F, Ovsenik M, et al. A controlled study of the functional and morphological characteristics of malocclusion in prematurely born subjects with low birthweight. Eur J Orthod 2014;36(1):114–20.

57. Taji SS, Seow WK. A literature review of dental erosion in children. Aust Dent J 2010;55:358–67 [systematic review].

58. Carvalho TS, Lussi A, Jaeggi T, et al. Erosive tooth wear in children. In: Lussi A, Ganss C, editors. Erosive tooth wear, vol. 25. Basel (Switzerland): Karger, Monogr Oral Sci; 2014. p. 262–78.

59. Corica A, Caprioglio A. Meta-analysis of the prevalence of tooth wear in primary dentition. Eur J Paediatr Dent 2014;15(4):385–8 [systematic review].

60. Lussi A, Jaeggi T. Dental erosion in children. In: Lussi A, Ganss C, editors. Dental erosion in childrenvol. 20. Basel (Switzerland): Karger, Monogr Oral Sci; 2006. p. 140–51.

61. Seow WK, Wan A. A controlled study of the morphometric changes in the primary dentition of pre-term, very-low-birthweight children. J Dent Res 2000; 79:63–9.

62. Fearne JM, Brook AH. Small primary tooth-crown size in low birthweight children. Early Hum Dev 1993;33:81–90.

63. Demarini S. Calcium and phosphorus nutrition in preterm infants. Acta Paediatr Suppl 2005;94(449):87–92.

64. Van den Oever HL, Versteegh FG, Thewessen EA, et al. Ciprofloxacin in preterm neonates: case report and review of the literature. Eur J Paediatr 1998;157: 843–5.

65. Seow WK, Humphrys C, Mahanonda R, et al. Dental eruption in low birthweight prematurely born children: a controlled study. Pediatr Dent 1988;10:39–42.

66. Seow WK. A study of the development of the permanent dentition in very low birthweight children. Pediatr Dent 1996;18:379–84.

67. Backstrom MC, Aine L, Maki R, et al. Maturation of primary and permanent teeth in preterm infants. Arch Dis Child Fetal Neonatal Ed 2000;83:F104–8.

68. Paulsson L, Bondemark L. Craniofacial morphology in prematurely born children. Angle Orthod 2009;79:276–83.

69. Molteni RA, Bumstread DH. Development and severity of palatal grooves in orally intubated newborns. Am J Dis Child 1986;140:357–9.

70. Paulsson L, Bondemark L, Soderfeldt B. A systematic review of the consequences of premature birth on palatal morphology, dental occlusion, tooth-crown dimensions and tooth maturity and eruption. Angle Orthod 2004;74: 269–79 [systematic review].

71. Proffit WR. The etiology of orthodontic problems. In: Proffit WR, editor. Contemporary orthodontics. St Louis (MO): Mosby Elsevier; 2007. p. 151–60.

72. Warren JJ, Bishara SE. Duration of nutritive and non-nutritive sucking behaviors and their effects on the dental arches in the primary dentition. Am J Orthod Dentofacial Orthop 2002;121:347–56.

73. Pinelli J, Symington A. Non-nutritive sucking for promoting physiologic stability and nutrition in preterm infants. Cochrane Database Syst Rev 2005;(4):CD001071. [systematic review].

74. Di Pietro JA, Cusson RM, Caughy MO, et al. Behavioral and physiologic effects of nonnutritive sucking during gavage feeding in preterm infants. Pediatr Res 1994;36(2):207.

75. Macey-Dare LV, Moles DR, Evans RD, et al. Long-term effect of neonatal endotracheal intubation on palatal form and symmetry in 8-11-year-old children. Eur J Orthod 1999;21:703–10.

76. Warren JJ, Slayton RL, Bishara SE, et al. Effects of non-nutritive sucking habits on occlusal characteristics in the mixed dentition. Pediatr Dent 2005;27(6): 445–50.
77. Dimberg L, Bondemark L, Soderfeldt B, et al. Prevalence of malocclusion traits and sucking habits among 3 year old children. Swed Dent J 2010;34(1):35–42.
78. Dimberg L, Lennartsson B, Soderfeldt B, et al. Malocclusions in children at 3 and 7 years of age: a longitudinal study. Eur J Orthod 2013;35(1):131–7.
79. Silva M, Manton D. Oral habits – part 1: the dental effects and management of nutritive and non-nutritive sucking. J Dent Child (Chic) 2014;81(3):133–9.
80. Silva M, Manton D. Oral habits – part 2: beyond nutritive and non-nutritive sucking. J Dent Child (chic) 2014;81(3):140–6.
81. Viggiano D, Fasano D, Monaco G, et al. Breast feeding, bottle feeding, and non-nutritive sucking; effects on occlusion in deciduous dentition. Arch Dis Child 2004;89:1121–3.
82. Sanchez-Molins M, Grau Carbo J, Lischeid Gaig C, et al. Comparative study of the craniofacial growth depending on the type of lactation received. Eur J Paediatr Dent 2010;11:87–92.
83. Romero CC, Scavone-Junior H, Garib DG, et al. Breast-feeding and non-nutritive sucking patterns related to the prevalence of anterior open bite in primary dentition. J Appl Oral Sci 2011;19:161–8.
84. American Academy of Pediatric Dentistry. Guideline on cares-risk assessment and management for infants, Child Adolescents. 2014. Clinical Guidelines. p. 141–5. Available at: www.aapd.org/media/Policies_Guidelines/G_cariesriskassessment.pdf. Accessed September 02, 2015.
85. American Academy of Pediatric Dentistry. Guideline on infant oral health care. 2014. Clinical Guidelines. p. 141–5. Available at: www.aapd.org/media/Policies_Guidelines/G_InfantOralHealthCare.pdf. Accessed September 02, 2015.
86. American Academy of Pediatric Dentistry. Guideline on management of dental patients with special health care needs. 2012. Clinical Guidelines. p. 161–6. Available at: www.aapd.org/media/Policies_Guidelines/G_SHCN.pdf. Accessed September 02, 2015.
87. Hurlbutt M, Young DA. A best practices approach to caries management. J Evid Based Dent Pract 2014;14(Suppl):77–86.
88. American Academy of Pediatric Dentistry. Policy on the dental home. Reference Manual. vol. 36(no.6). 2014/2015. 2012. p. 24–5. Available at: www.aapd.org/media/Policies_Guidelines/P_DentalHome.pdf. Accessed September 02, 2015.
89. Ramos-Gomez FJ, Crall J, Gansky SA, et al. Caries risk assessment appropriate for the age 1 visit (infants and toddlers). J Calif Dent Assoc 2007;35(10): 687–702.
90. Ramos-Gomez FJ, Ng MW. Into the future: keeping healthy teeth caries free: pediatric CAMBRA protocols. J Calif Dent Assoc 2011;39(10):723–33.
91. Twetman S. Caries prevention with fluoride toothpaste in children: an update. Eur Arch Paediatr Dent 2009;10(3):162–7.
92. Neves BG, Farah A, Lucas E, et al. Are pediatric medicines risk factors for dental caries and dental erosion? Community Dent Health 2010;27:46–51.
93. Zhan L, Cheng J, Chang P, et al. Effects of xylitol wipes on cariogenic bacteria and caries in young children. J Dent Res 2012;91(Suppl 7):85S–90S.
94. Steinberg BJ, Hilton IV, Iida H, et al. Oral health and dental care during pregnancy. Dent Clin North Am 2013;57:195–210.
95. Chou R, Cantor A, Zakher B, et al. Prevention of dental caries in children younger than 5 years old: systematic review to update the US Preventive

Services Task Force Recommendation. Rockville (MD): Agency for Healthcare Research and quality US; 2014. Report No.: 12-05170-EF-1.

96. Twetman S, Dhar V. Evidence of effectiveness of current therapies to prevent and treat early childhood caries. Pediatr Dent 2015;37(3):246–53 [systematic review].
97. Slayton RL. Clinical decision-making for caries management in children: an update. Pediatr Dent 2015;37(2):106–10 [systematic review].
98. Wan AKL, Seow WK, Purdie DM, et al. A longitudinal study of Streptococcus mutans colonization in infants after tooth eruption. J Dent Res 2003;82:504–8.
99. Schroth RJ, Smith PJ, Whalen JC, et al. Prevalence of caries among preschool-aged children in a northern Manitoba community. J Can Dent Assoc 2005;71(1). 27a-f.
100. Bader JD. Casein phosphopeptide-amorphous calcium phosphate shows promise for preventing caries. Evid Based Dent 2010;11(1):11–2.
101. Cochrane NJ, Reynolds EC. Caclium phosphopetides – mechanisms of action and evidence for clinical efficacy. Adv Dent Res 2012;24(2):41–7.
102. Zhou C, Zhang D, Bai Y, et al. Casein phosphopeptide-amorphous calcium phosphate remineralization of primary teeth early enamel lesions. J Dent 2014;42(1):21–9.
103. Tinanoff N, Coll JA, Dhar V, et al. Evidence-based update of pediatric dental restorative procedures: preventive strategies. J Clin Pediatr Dent 2015;39(3): 193–7.
104. Bhujel N, Duggal M, Munyombwe T, et al. The effect of premature extraction of primary teeth on the subsequent need for orthodontic treatment. Eur Arch Paediatr Dent 2014;15(6):393–400.
105. Donly KJ, Garcia-Godoy F. The use of resin-based composite in children: an update. Pediatr Dent 2015;37(2):136–43 [systematic review].
106. Seale NS, Randall R. The use of stainless steel crowns: a systematic literature review. Pediatr Dent 2015;37(2):147–62 [systematic review].
107. Waggoner WF. Restoring primary anterior teeth: updated for 2014. Pediatr Dent 2015;37(2):163–70 [systematic review].
108. Kreulen CM, Van't Spijker A, Rodriguez JM, et al. Systematic review of the prevalence of tooth wear in children and adolescents. Caries Res 2010;44(2): 151–9 [systematic review].
109. Levy FM, Magalhaes AC, Gomes MF, et al. The erosion and abrasion-inhibiting effect of TiF(4) and NaF varnishes and solutions on enamel in vitro. Int J Paediatr Dent 2012;22(1):11–6.
110. Lussi A, Carvalho TS. The future of fluorides and other protective agents in erosion prevention. Caries Res 2015;49(Suppl 1):18–29.

Index

Note: Page numbers of article titles are in **boldface** type.

A

Alzheimer disease, clinical presentation of, 709–710
    definition and epidemiology of, 709
    dental management of, 713
    medical management of, 712–713
    patient management in, 713–714
    stages of, 710–711
    treatment modifications in, 714–715
Americans with Disabilities Act, See also *Disabilities*., **627–647**
    Amendments Act of 2008, 629
    communication and, 631–632
    curb ramps and, 631
    definition of "developmental disability" and, 628–629
    definition of "disability" and, 628, 629
    dental offices and, 629
    disability access claims and, 632–633
    Equal Employment Opportunity Commission and, 629
    local government ordinances and, 632
    requirements of, local governments and, 631–632
    US Supreme Court and, 632
Anesthesia, general, dental treatment of IDD patients under, 595
Aphasia, 698
Autism Spectrum disorder, DSM-5 current terminology for, 641–642
    vaccine injuries in, judicial proceedings in, 642

B

Biomedical ethics, 634–636
    autonomy and, 635–636
    distributive justice and, 636
    nonmaleficence and, 635
Bite block (mouth prop) foam, 580–581, 600, 601, 602
Bleeding, medications increasing, 719
Bridge, hygienic, for IDD patients, 580–581, 600, 601, 602
Brush, interdental, 598, 599
    triple-headed, 598, 599

C

California Welfare and Institutions Code, 640
Caries, checking for, 582, 584
Cerebral palsy, classification of, 643–644, 645

Dent Clin N Am 60 (2016) 757–763
http://dx.doi.org/10.1016/S0011-8532(16)30042-8
0011-8532/16/$ – see front matter

X

Moving?

Make sure your subscription moves with you!

To notify us of your new address, find your **Clinics Account Number** (located on your mailing label above your name), and contact customer service at:

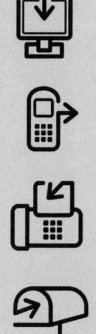

Email: journalscustomerservice-usa@elsevier.com

800-654-2452 (subscribers in the U.S. & Canada)
314-447-8871 (subscribers outside of the U.S. & Canada)

Fax number: 314-447-8029

Elsevier Health Sciences Division
Subscription Customer Service
3251 Riverport Lane
Maryland Heights, MO 63043

*To ensure uninterrupted delivery of your subscription, please notify us at least 4 weeks in advance of move.

ELSEVIER

Printed and bound by CPI Group (UK) Ltd, Croydon, CR0 4YY

03/10/2024

01040393-0004